SEX, LOVE, & WORTH

How I Survived
College Without Sex
and Discovered Love

ANTHONY SIMON

ISBN: 978-0-578-23020-7

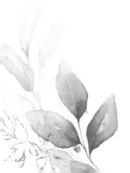

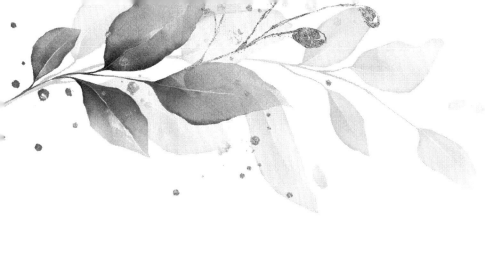

To my future spouse:
I love you with all my body
I love you with all my mind
I love you with all my soul
I love you with all my heart
Nothing will ever separate us apart

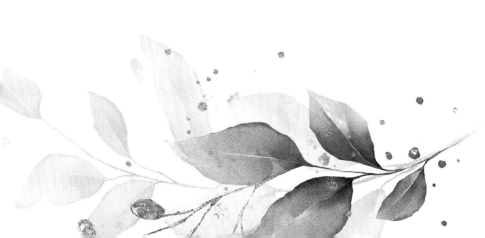

A SPECIAL NOTE TO THE READER

To the Seeking Lover,

You went on a quest looking for true love
Hoping to find your one and only beloved
You left with a heart full of hope
Never knowing you'd come back to mope
You thought you caught the prize everyone looked upon
Months later you found out you were cheated on
You took a risk to prove people wrong
Tsk, tsk, you ended up reading this sad song
I understand you were severely rejected
I understand your body was merely objected
You poured out your heart
But your significant other didn't do their part
They used you just for sex
And made everything so dang complex
They said it was love so you gave them your full trust
Turns out it was nothing but dirty ol' lust
Your heart felt so stranded
Nothing was enough, even being so candid
I bet you never knew
You could ever feel this blue
Left with shame and low self-esteem, you put on a mask
Your mom noticed and began to ask

You turned out to be nothing but a useless slave"
You began to have a hardened heart
All you wanted to do was press rewind and restart
A bad hand was all that was dealt
At the end of the day, emotional rejection was all you felt
Your parents failed and didn't do their part
You father divorced your mother, tearing your little heart
At the age of two this tragedy left a big stain
How could you not point the finger and blame?
I can't justify the unspeakable pains that happened to you
Nobody understands, not even a few
People don't realize that you're so fragile
They don't see your heart, just a masked smile
I know you feel like nobody cares if you even live
But please, open your heart and allow me to give
It's too soon to take your life away
Can you just give me a chance and say
"I'm done trying to rhyme
I promise, this heartbreak will be your very last time."

Your relationship coach,
Anthony Simon

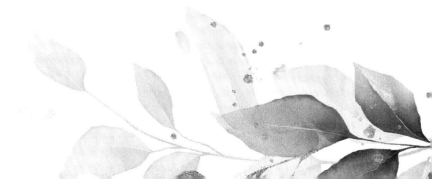

CONTENTS

PART 2: FINDING LOVE & WORTH

PART 3: BUILDING LOVE & WORTH

PART 4: GIVING LOVE & WORTH

INTRODUCTION
Yo, Broski! Read This

S ex is amazing.

Whoops. I didn't mean to open the book like that.

What I meant to say is . . . stop settling in your relationships.

Allow me to introduce myself. I'm Anthony, and I'm a regular twenty-two-year-old guy, a former college athlete, and a virgin by choice who is proud of his decision. Yes, it's true—regular, athletic college guys who are also virgins still exist.

It might sound counterintuitive, but remaining pure through college has given me a lot of important insight into sex, love, and worth that I have used to improve both my own life and the lives of others I work with as a love and relationship coach. This is the stuff nobody ever talks about—the secrets about sex, standards, relationships, forming intimate bonds, finding your truest worth, and, most importantly, meeting love face-to-face and understanding what it means to love and be loved to your fullest capacity.

Wait, wait. Before you close this book saying, "This goofy dweeb has no experience in dating. He's just stalling and wasting my time. He's never actually had intimate connections or slept with beautiful women. Why should I listen to him?" just hear me out for a moment.

If you know anything about student athletes and public school universities in California, you know there's plenty of temptation and opportunities to hook up and get into relationships. I mean, there's the special-invite parties from frats and sororities, bars, late-night exchanges with other athletes, classes, banquets, and social gatherings attended by lot of horny males and females thirsting for love and intimacy to cover their wounds and find a Band-Aid solution for their sense of worth and value.

So, with temptation everywhere, why would this goofy dweeb want to wait until marriage? If you think it's a religious manipulation, insecurity, fear, self-doubt, lack of opportunity, or even lack of interest in women, guess again. You may be surprised by the answer.

But before you even read on, let's make sure this is the right book for you. These are deep, life-altering life hacks for relationships that will change your mindset and prepare you for a new chapter of your life to unfold. So you've got to be ready for it.

This book isn't for you if you're not looking to give me your full heart and mind. What I'm going to do is go deep . . . DEEP into the depths of your soul. I'm going to wake you up and show you love is possible. You *CAN* find someone who will truly love you for you. Do any of these bullets describe you?

THIS BOOK IS FOR YOU IF YOU'RE:

- Lowering your standards and giving pieces of your heart, body, or soul to someone who's selfishly using you so you can *potentially* get him/her to stay, love, or value you for less than you know you're worth.
- Trying to understand why she or he left you after you've given them literally everything.
- A college or high school student (single, dating, a virgin, not a virgin, religious, not religious) who has lost hope and feels there's no true, selfless, pure love out there anymore.

- Looking to prevent relationships ending bitterly, getting cheated on, dumped, or rejected.
- Having casual sex in college just for fun or because you're bored, and wondering why you can't connect.
- Wondering why you're still attracted to broken relationships that aren't right for you, feel something is missing, feel bored, or are not happy in any relationship you get into.
- Trying to heal from a traumatic past such as rejection, being cheated on, abuse, being fatherless/motherless, or neglect that's haunting you whenever you get into a relationship.
- Searching for your sense of worth, identity and self-esteem after losing yourself to a stubborn heartbreak that left you emptier than when you started.

At one point in my life, I checked off almost all of those bullet points. I'm excited to share with you my experiences with dating, love, and the lessons I've learned from not only my mistakes, but those of others too.

HOW TO READ THIS BOOK

WAIT! Did you hear that? Hey, hey, quiet down. I need your full attention. Sssshhhhh, be quiet.

My heart is telling me to ask you for a quick favor before letting you in on my big secret. It's saying, "Anthony, don't trust everyone. At least have the reader earn your trust first. You're always so eager to share."

I don't want you making too much noise, so I'm going to need you to keep a promise for me. The only way I can gain your trust with my big secret is by getting you to do this tiny favor for me.

STOP! Look to the right and left, over your shoulder, to make sure nobody is around. I don't want just anyone doing me this tiny favor.

What? What's that you ask? No, no, don't be silly now. I'm not asking for your bank account; I'm asking for something more valuable. . . .

Again, I'm asking for the deepest parts of your heart. (And no, to you extreme people, we are not getting married. I'm speaking figuratively, trying to be smooth.) The tiny favor is to promise me that you're going to read this entire introduction, and the first two chapters of the book diligently and focused.

As you're reading, I'm asking you to give me permission to enter into your heart. Open your mind and heart to what I have to say. Do so by getting your favorite pen and journal and reflecting on the questions, key points, and action steps at the end of every chapter.

The quality of your life is determined by the quality of questions you ask yourself. There will be questions and action steps at the end of each chapter guiding you through each part to ultiamtely give you the tools to find uncondtional love and sustaining happiness. I want you to be honest with your past, present and future self by getting a special journal and thoroughly answering them. The more honest and detailed you are with your responses, the greater results you'll receive.

If you don't do these things, I can't give you the secret. I'm giving you my heart, so I expect to get yours as well. It's part of the deal. Can we make a promise on that? This introduction and the first two chapters set the tone for the whole book. They are highly recommended to read. (Yeah, I hope I didn't sound like your professor. I'm still only twenty-two.)

WHAT YOU WILL LEARN

WE'RE GOING TO GO ON A JOURNEY, BABY! I'm just excited for you. Seriously. I'm actually smiling right now as I'm writing this. I don't think you understand what's going to hit you (yes, physically too) and how much joy you're going to get. You will probably cry (yes, you "tough" men out there too). There may be moments you may feel the need to jump out of your chair screaming, "LET'S GO, BABY!" This is going to be a roller coaster ride full of adventure, smiles, and tears of hope and healing too, so make sure to get comfortable and grab a box of tissue.

Some of the greatest secrets about forming intimate relationships with others and finding your true identity and worth aren't being talked about anymore. Why? Well, because they are secrets, and if you know anything about secrets, the selfish world loves to hide them from you. In this book, you'll be learning the secrets, if—yes, *IF*—you will decide to change and are sick and tired of being sick and tired, hopeless, reckless, or even wondering if there's more to sex, love, and your worth than you think. Hold on. Before I reveal them to you, you and I have to go through the boring part of making sure you're not going to waste my time or yours. Some of the secrets I'm going to talk about include:

- The shameless naked truth about sex through psychology, science, and nature
- The secrets to getting into the best relationship of your life and finding true, loyal love
- The secrets to love, being seen, and being loved by anyone despite your past or present
- The loveable laws of finding lovely love ;)
- How to find your *full* identity, *full* worth, and *full* love, and gift it to someone who understands the value
- Why some relationships work and others fail, and how to test a relationship to see if it will last
- How to identify and destroy the beautiful lies that are stopping you from falling in love, finding your truest worth, and becoming the best version of yourself—physically, intellectually, mentally, emotionally, and spiritually.

WHY LISTEN TO ME?

Sex is amazing. Duhhhhhh. How many more times do I have to say it?

All right, you're not convinced. You see, I don't want to be the boring person who tells you about how I graduated from the University of California, Davis, with degrees in communications (B.A.) and biopsychology (B.S) and now travel throughout the U.S. giving relationship talks and motivational speeches. To me, education is cool and all, but I'm all about experiences—good and bad. Yes, that means failures. I have failed countless times, which is why I am writing a book on this so you don't fail too. You remember the first book I wrote? Well, for those of you that don't, it's titled *Life's Greatest Gift: P.A.I.N.* All of my pain came because I didn't know my identity, worth, and value. I mistakenly settled, giving away pieces of my heart and lowering my standards so I could potentially heal my wounds. It didn't work, and I only dug myself in a deeper hole. After intense reflection and guidance by the greatest relationship coaches in the world, I now write books and travel all over the United States teaching people how to live in sustaining happiness and unconditional love in their relationships.

I genuinely care for you. I really suffered a lot and I don't want you to go through what I went through because it was really painful. You can learn through my failures. I want to save you time in the dating world and help you to find sustaining happiness and love, especially if you're in high school, college, or post-grad. I've seen too many relationships end poorly (especially mine), and they happen when we're young, because we don't know any better.

Don't believe me? Then why do more than 50 percent of marriages end in divorce? Why do the majority of relationships last no more than a couple months? Why do the statistics only show that our newer generation is becoming more depressed, lonely, rejected, anxious, isolated, obese, and lacking in identity, purpose, vision, and passion? You don't have to use your brain to recognize that relationships in college, and especially in high school, only last for a quick-fused, passionate several months, leaving your self-esteem emptier than when you started. Anything past that stage begins to die down because most relationships were based only on feelings, lust, insecurities, lack of knowledge about your worth, or even lack of identity. It's no wonder your significant other got bored and decided to leave or cheat on you with someone else.

I understand that you and I are born with a nature that's wicked and we cultivate that darkness the more that hatred is inflicted. I understand that you were born being rejected and not perfectly loved from the start of your life, which led to bad outcomes. You may have been looking for love in all the wrong areas.

You gave it all but it wasn't enough . . . it didn't work out. You're deeply wounded and bleeding at the depths of your heart—your soul. Your initial reaction is to try and cover it up with another relationship. You use it as a bandage or towel until it stops bleeding, but it won't stop bleeding. Why? It's simple: Because you weren't just born to be loved and to love; you were born to be loved and to love at your *fullest* potential. You were born to be seen for who you authentically are. When authentic, pure love is not received, it leaves a deep internal wound that most of us can't see. Someone who has had his wounds and scars exposed has to help you see them too. Allow me to be the bridge to turn your painful scars to sacred scars.

You may be living a comfortable, beautiful lie in your current relationship, where you're being used and devalued without even realizing it because you don't even know your own worth. Well, I'm going to shine the glamourous, raw, liberating truth on to those comfortable, entertaining, love-stealing, beautiful lies.

Or maybe you're on the opposite end of the spectrum . . . you've decided to wait for the right person. You're in a season of singleness that feels like an eternity and you're tempted to lower your standards because everyone else around you looks happy and feels great on the outside but are suffering in their inner selves. Don't give up just yet. Don't fall into the trap like I did. There is hope. I know you may feel alone, rejected, and abandoned, but you're not. Don't listen to those beautiful lies—they will only eat your soul day by day. I almost ended my life because of them. Don't allow your fear of being alone trick you into lowering your standards and sabotaging your value.

I get it, you may be in a relationship right now that you're not fully satisfied with. You may be looking for love in what you think is the right place only to find out it was a mirage. You may have experienced abuse, or maybe several traumatizing relationships that left you bitter, angry, and resentful. You gave everything selflessly, expecting nothing in return. But wait, you did receive something when you were least expecting it: abuse, manipulation, trauma, heartbreak, physical pain, emotional pain, a crushed spirit, self-hatred, depression, or even a loss of your own identity.

Whatever stage you're in right now, please allow me to inform and inspire you to live out the four-step process to finding pure love, your fullest worth, and a happiness that overflows from your heart to another's heart. This four-step process is the life secret to finding a transforming love that is literally out of this world and transcends any love you've ever experienced.

1. Part I: Seeking Love and Worth—Mind and Heart Education
2. Part II: Finding Love and Worth—Mind and Heart Transformation
3. Part III: Building Love and Worth—Behavior Modification
4. Part IV: Giving Love and Worth—Sexual Liberation

There is no time like this season you're in. This is the best and only time of your life where you can bring every dream into fruition, discover just how precious you are, and find a joyful, shame-free sex life. You can never get this time back. Start working now before regret comes unexpectedly knocking at your door and breaking in to steal every ounce of happiness you saved in your half-full cup thinking it's full.

Let me tell you, the truth will always come out. It's only a matter of time until you find out if you are really happy in your current relationship, and if that guy or girl is worth your time to stay with or pursue someone else. This book will help reveal that truth faster so you can claim a life you deserve but are being robbed of.

WHY I CHOSE TO WRITE THIS BOOK

Please. You've got to understand something. I'm speaking heart-to-heart right now. I keep it real. Whether you accept it as the truth or not, I'm not going to settle and give you something less than the truth because you deserve nothing but the truth.

I wasn't going to write this book. There were so many doubts and fears I had about publishing it. "What will people think?" "Will this ruin my image as a speaker?" "What if people make fun of me?" "Will I ever be looked at the same?" "Is this actually going to touch people's hearts?" "Will people think I'm bragging or that I'm saying I'm better than others for being a virgin or sharing my stories?" "Will the people in my inner circle criticize me?" "Will I lose friends or respect from others by sharing my testimony?" "Will people reject or accept me?" Blah, blah, blah! All these fears and doubts took a toll on me and I waited for the right time to publish this book. I had thought about publishing it last year but my worries got the best of me for a while. In the end, I decided it didn't matter. I may be the greatest fool for publishing this book, but it's worth the risk to potentially gain an inch of your heart and bring it to the light. If anything, now is the time to be bold and courageous, because so many aren't.

I didn't do this for pity, Instagram likes, reviews, praise, or my own self-righteous glory. That's not where my heart is with this all. I didn't write this book just to write another book because it looks good on my resume or makes money. I didn't want to just be another person who talks about sex, love, relationships, finding your self-worth, and dating claiming to know it all. The fact is, I don't know it all. That's not why I wrote this book. No, I wrote this book because I've failed many times in my life, as I keep reiterating. I wrote this book because, as I gave talks, I've seen moms crying and pouring out their heart to me for their children who were in toxic relationships. I've known fathers who committed suicide because they married the wrong person and got cheated on. I've heard of countless relationships that failed because they couldn't connect. I've talked to countless kids who don't know who they are and how much they are worth. And I've heard far too many regrets.

If I were writing just *another self-help book on love* I would've put together a basic book telling you what you *want* to hear and not what you *need* to hear. But I couldn't stand trusting the self-proclaiming and self-electing "dating gurus" who just left me disappointed and more restless just so they could steal my money, time, and attention.

These self-made leaders claimed to have the truth yet they still had bitter lives. They were living beautiful lies, which they knew and felt, but refused to change. I was tired of wolves in sheep's clothing—people who gave empty promises and somewhat temporary, satisfying results. I wanted nothing but the truth and ONLY the truth. I wanted the best results. The. ABSOLUTE. Best.

It couldn't just be the truth; it had to have come from a pure heart and be received with love. So many people would give the truth in exchange for their own selfish motives, desires, or pleasures. I would feel used and not feel loved, so I wouldn't be able to accept their message as the truth.

My goal is not to condemn, judge, label, manipulate, or point a finger at you. Nope. My job is to return the love I have received in my life back to you in a gentle way. I got it the tough way and I want you to get it the tender way. I don't want you feeling used. This is costing me more than it is helping me. I sacrificed a lot just so I could *potentially* see you happy.

Did you catch that?

I sacrificed a lot just so I could *POTENTIALLY* see you happy.

You know what pains me the most? I have met countless women and men thirsting for the truth about sex, intimacy in relationships, worth, identity, and pure, unconditional love. So many of them have the right motives to find authentic love, but many come home heartbroken, depressed, or in despair because they didn't realize they have been programmed by society and the beautiful lies our culture tells us about love. Heck, some don't even come home. Some end their lives. It makes me shed tears just thinking about right now. If it weren't for a dear parent and her daughter, whom I hold close to my heart, this book would've never been written.

I found the equation to love and be loved at your fullest potential. I found the equation to life-sustaining happiness. I don't just talk about it, I live it. If you know anything about me, you know I'm a joyful person who smiles a lot and genuinely loves his life. (It's my slogan, *Love Your Life*). You know it's real because you won't only *see* it, but you'll *feel* it in me. These aren't my words, but what others have been saying about me. I've been told that my joy is contagious. Everyone always asks, "Anthony, how did you become so happy? I know you're not faking it. What drives you? What makes you get up every day so fully alive? What's the secret? How are you able to love so well? When did you change? What happened to you, man? Who was it?" They assume I'm sleeping with women, but when I tell them, "Guess again, I'm a virgin!" they pause what they're doing and are in disbelief. Then they ask me, "What is it then?"

I'm about to show you what it is right now. Just promise me you'll read this book in order and actually finish it. I know so many people who buy books and they just collect dust. Don't be one of those people. Be one of the top 1 percent who commits and finishes because they're driven by their actions, not only words, to find unconditional love.

I knew I had the secret magic potion equation to love that many thought they had. I had found the pearl that was hidden in the depths of my own house, locked in a treasure chest. After several years of proper thought and intense contemplation, I gathered all the evidence to write this book. But it was really the encounters with this beautiful, loving mother that made me actually decide to share my pearl with the world instead of being selfish and keeping it to myself because of fear or doubt.

This pearl is the secret to why I get up every day smiling, saying, "I LOVE MY LIFE, BABY! I FOUND MY DREAM GIRL! LET'S GO!"

After years of suffering, I have found the truth about love, relationships, sex, and the hidden buried secrets to being loved and loving at my fullest potential.

Are you ready for them?

It's in my essence to share with you the secrets to getting into the best relationships of your life. I can't promise you anything but the truth. What you do with the truth is up to you.

You see, many say they are ready but I'm disappointed to see they've lied to me. Can you handle the truth? Many think they can, but when it's told to them, they get frustrated or mad.

Are you ready? Remember the promise we made in exchange for the secret? Well, let's follow through on that. See you on the next page.

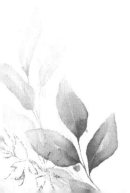

PART 1
Seeking Love
& Worth

1

Expectations of Sex

Sex.

How good can sex actually be? Let's find out.

Here's what some said:

"Sex doesn't equal love. It's a lie. Sex isn't casual. I'm sick of being in a new relationship every month. I can't fall in love anymore. Screw women, I don't need them. They are boring and they don't get me."

"Nobody ever taught me how a man should love me. I was adopted, with no father in my life. I completely lost myself having sex with over fifty men. I don't feel like I have any value anymore, Anthony. I'm not worth anything. I'm just a piece of meat being tossed around."

"I've slept with over one hundred women and I am just bored of having sex. It has no meaning to me anymore. Sex is just casual."

"I wish I had the willpower you have. I can't focus and it takes so much of my time. I'm a slave to this desire of sex that I don't want and leaves me emptier, more broken, used, and confused."

"I didn't know. Nobody taught me how sacred sex was. I didn't have parents educating me on sex. I just figured it was like the movies. You do it and fall in love. I was wrong. I lost myself and cried after having sex because it was nothing like the world told me it was. What is love? Where do I find love?"

"I'm all used up. Why do I deserve love after everyone I slept with? There aren't any good men left and even if there were, why would they want me? Can I really change? If I do change, is it worthwhile? Is love even worth the risk? I feel overwhelmed with shame. I'm a slave to pleasure."

"I don't feel any connection in the bedroom. I have to fake my emotions to please them . . . it doesn't help that I don't feel good enough and insecure too. What's wrong with me?"

"I used to say, 'Waiting doesn't apply to me since I'm dating the one I'm going to marry.' When we got married, I saw how sex covered up problems in our lives we didn't know we had. Now, they are magnified in our marriage and we're both suffering because of it."

". . . Go out and experience so you're prepared for your marriage day and you won't feel shy or embarrassed. Seems believable at first until you actually get married. Man, I'm more embarrassed now knowing it's not just her in the bedroom."

"I can't see my daughter living the life I lived. I had sex in the past and I still can't get rid of the memories from the past men. It affected my marriage and now I'm seeing my daughter go through the same mistakes I made. I hope she could just come back and realize it's a dead end. I didn't have parents tell me right from wrong . . . all I wanted to be was the parent to her that I never had."

"I thought it was just a casual hookup. We had sex, and three years later I still can't get her out of my mind. Why am I still attached and thinking about her?"

"The world said having sex would make me a man. At first it's fun, but the more women I pulled, the more I lost myself. It was a trap. I regret even listening in the first place. I shouldn't have listened and now I'm suffering. It's not worth it, man. I hate my life sitting in this jail cell."

"I just wanted to get rid of my virginity. Everyone was doing it; what's the harm? I was wrong. I don't know who I am anymore and I just want to take my life away. There are some days I come close."

"I wanted to be experienced. I wanted to test the car before I bought it so I could guarantee falling in love with it. Didn't work out and now I feel like I gave away my money for a broken car."

". . . I don't want to lose him. He won't love me unless I have sex. He's been so nice to me; I owe it to him. So, I gave it to him. I was great the first couple months until he got bored and cheated on me. I feel reduced to an animal. I can't believe it. This is so painful and I don't know what to do."

". . . 'We're already in love with each other, why should I wait?' I'm married and now I see why I should've waited. Some days I feel like I'm sleeping with my ex."

"I'm so lost. Nobody is out there for me. How come I can't connect with anyone even if I have sex with them? Maybe I'm turning gay?"

"I keep pleasing men and giving pieces of my body to them but they never stay with me. Am I the problem? Am I good enough? I must not be skinny enough."

"I hate it. I don't know why I can't be committed to one girl, man. I just don't get hard anymore."

"I got bored. She was too boring for me. Sex is getting boring, dude; it's not a big deal."

"I gave my virginity to him hoping he would stay with me. Now I'm stuck with someone who's just using me for my body and treating me like trash. I want to leave but I can't. I feel trapped. Please help."

"I thought we were just friends with benefits. I don't know how, but I caught feelings. Sex complicated everything and I feel so heartless."

"I've been married for ten years now and I still think of those women when I sleep with my wife."

LOVE IS LOVE, RIGHT?

Soooooo . . . I guess sex is not that good . . . right?

Wrong.

It breaks my heart hearing people's bitter, dark, frustrated, suppressed stories about their experiences with sex, forming intimate

3

relationships, finding their authentic worth, and finding pure love. Many people have sincere desires and intentions to find love, but so many have bitter experiences that are either known or unknown. Why? Why do so many people fail? And how can you avoid falling into the same traps everyone else does? Keep reading.

> **Many people have sincere desires and intentions to find love, but so many have bitter experiences that are either known or unknown.**

My goal isn't to scare you or get rid of your sexual desires, but to help you master those desires for the sake of authentic love.

If love were love, you wouldn't hear countless broken relationship stories like these. There has to be some universal truths about what love and sex are and aren't.

NO, I'M NOT ANTI-SEX

I'll say it again: I'm not anti-sex. Surprise!

I love sex. You love sex. Animals love sex. We all love sex because we all want love and happiness. The only problem is most of us don't know exactly what sex or love is. We just suck up whatever the world tells us and form unrealistic expectations about sex that are completely false, with empty promises. This is why so many people are lowering their standards. It starts with a heartbreak and, without realizing it, you gradually and subtly lower your standards, convincing yourself this is how life is supposed to be.

It's time for the truth. The truth that will set you free from all the lies.

The problem is, there are so many voices in the world giving partial truths and even straight-up lies about what sex is and what it isn't. What love is and what love isn't. Who you are and who you aren't. You can see this because you read the experiences above. It's clear that most of us fall into the same traps as my friends, inner circle, and people I've encountered through speaking have fallen into. We really don't know how to have unifying, bonding, and intimate relationships through sex, or even the proper way to love and cultivate relationships that flourish, not diminish. Of no fault of our own, we cheapen and commercialize sex as less than what it truly is by not understanding the value and purpose it serves.

> *Most relationships fail because of a lack of knowledge of what sex is, what love is, and how much we're worth.*

Most relationships fail because of a lack of knowledge of what sex is, what love is, and how much we're worth. We don't know how we're supposed to view it, and why. Sexual understanding is not just about behavior modification. Rather, it is about heart and mind transformation, which comes from heart and mind revelation. With this, you have sexual liberation and can understand how good your love life can really be.

Instead of having someone tell you, "Don't do this and do that," you need to hear, "This is why listening matters in the first place." As you continue reading, just be open to the *whys* and you will respect why I chose to remain a virgin, even through college.

I know what you're thinking. "Oh, he's just scared to get a girl pregnant or catch a disease. He's anti-sex and doesn't like women, or never had any temptation. He never got into any relationships or even experienced failure. He must not understand anything about safe sex, the cycle, or any of that. He's ignorant, living in a cave from 350 B.C. He's probably one of those religious, judgmental kids who was manipulated to act this way out of fear or doubt. He's just trying to condemn me, guilt-trip me, or manipulate me into changing my life. Do you even have a girl now, dude? Results speak for themselves." Whoa, whoa, dude. Simmer down now, horsey, simmer down.

Although I'm not a baboon with a caveman stick, my blood brother Christopher tells me I have a tendency to act like a monkey. (Keep reading, I'm curious to see what you think.) I assure you I am no judgmental caveman. And I'm definitely no condemning prude trying to shove a delusional opinion down your throat. I'm just a dude who's trying to share a manly man's experiences and advice on love, sex, forming intimate relationships, and worth. This will help you find your own worth, and guide you toward a life where you aren't just existing, but truly living—living life abundantly and fully alive through authentic, pure love.

So before you judge me and start thinking I'm judging you, putting you down, or even assuming I'm saying I'm better than you, just open your heart and mind and please give me a chance. Point a finger at me and three more are pointing back at you. (Try it right now and you'll see what I mean. I'm full of witty jokes. Get used to it!) You and I can agree that there is always more we can learn on a subject, no matter how much we may already know. We can never be masters at a topic. So, I want you to learn from my unique perspective—a dude's perspective on sex, love, and worth. You always hear a ton of women talking about sex, love, and worth, but tell me, have you heard about it from a guy your age? Let alone one who's a virgin and knows how to articulate his feelings into words?

It's easy to get tired of hearing about the diseases, the unwed pregnancy rates, and the condemning, negative, manipulative, sheltered comments. If you're ready for a different, positive approach about the gift of sex and love, and how great it is actually meant to be, then keep reading with that desire in mind.

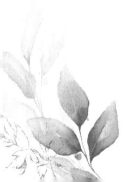

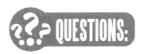 **QUESTIONS:**

1. Have any relationships ever failed? What did you learn from them?
2. Can you relate to any of the quotes above? How do you view sex? What is sex to you?
3. How badly do you desire love and to be seen? Are you willing to work for the best relationship?

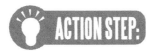 **ACTION STEP:**

1. Grab a journal and your favorite pen and answer/complete all the questions and action steps at the end of every chapter. Remember, this is a journey you're taking with me and I encourage you to email me your questions or revelations every chapter at coachanthonysimon@gmail.com

2

Dude, You Didn't Smash?

"This can't be happening. Are you serious? Is this real? Am I dreaming? Did this really just happen to me?"

I couldn't believe what I was seeing as a senior in high school. I had finally found my very first love after looking for so long. Katie Star (not her real name) was the star cheerleader and captain of her soccer team, making her one of the most popular girls at her school. Even though she was involved in many school activities, she was well known for her attractive body, face, and personality. She was the perfect blonde-haired person with green-blue eyes. Every guy was trying to get with her and every girl was trying to be just like her. These attributes fascinated us all, but what caught us by surprise was that she was still playing the game called "waiting until marriage to have sex." Katie Star was arguably the hottest virgin by choice you would've met in our area.

Making the conscious decision to remain a virgin for her future husband, she played hard-to-get because she knew her value, identity, and worth.

Making the conscious decision to remain a virgin for her future husband, she played hard-to-get because she knew her value, identity, and worth. Many people asked her out but got rejected because she knew they were just trying to take her virginity to become a "man." This showed me she didn't just want any guy . . . she wanted *THE* guy.

She carried herself proudly, knowing she carried the full package— looks, body, status, personality, and power. I say power because she still had her V-card, which made her carefully select who she wanted in her life.

People envied her because she was still in first place, proudly carrying her trophy that said, "I'm still a virgin and I'm proud of it. I'm waiting to have sex with my future husband to have the best relationship and give my full self to him." Her parents taught her that we lived in a culture that no longer prized sexual purity. "Saving sex for marriage" had fallen out of style and didn't exist anymore. Despite being seen as unhealthy, crazy, absurd, and even a delusional prude, she continued holding the trophy in her hands, telling everyone by her actions, "I'm still playing the game."

Katie and I went to different schools and she still caught my attention. I knew she was special because she wasn't looking for just any relationship; she was looking for *THE* relationship. I wanted to be with her as I had also made the conscious decision to remain pure in mind, body, spirit, and soul. One day, I found the courage within myself to ask her out. SHE SAID YES! We dated for a couple months and I couldn't believe it. I'd "scored" a smoking-hot date and everyone knew it.

Months passed by and she was beginning to fall in love with me. I took her out to eat one day at a fancy restaurant and explained to her how I'm waiting to have sex until marriage. She seemed on board but her body language said otherwise.

I took her home and as I dropped her off, she looked at me, winked, and said in a seductive voice, "So we're not going to have fun tonight? I thought you knew my parents were out of town, and you told me to dress up."

My mind was blown. I really loved this girl. My hormones kicked in but I remembered what I'd promised myself—I still wanted to play the game with her. Despite wanting to have sex, I did not want to do anything physical with her until I got to know who she truly was emotionally and spiritually. I told her, "Katie, although you're tempting me, I respect you too much to have sex with you right now. I want to show you that I'm seriously committed to getting to know you first, not your body." I don't know what changed in her, but she looked at me like I was unhealthy, crazy, absurd, and even a delusional prude who was stupid and out of this world. I remember she said, "Oh, I was just joking. Don't be silly. Hey, I'm feeling tired anyway and I'll see you next week. I had a really good time tonight. Thank you for everything."

I knew she didn't understand why I was still waiting, knowing we both were comfortable and liked each other. I tried to explain to her in more detail, but she said she was "too tried" for deep talk right now. Instead, she said a quick goodnight to me.

One day, school ended and I was in the locker room getting dressed for my high school basketball game. One of my friends interrupted me and said, "Last night, I went to a party and some dude got with Katie Star and had sex with her. I didn't believe it until I heard the guy tell one of his friends, 'DUDE! I just had sex with Katie Star. I took her virginity. I'm the real man now.' The other guy said, 'DANG, MAN! What a score, dude! Wish I could've too. You know, sharing is caring.'"

My body and face turned numb and I could not feel my heart. I just didn't believe this was happening to me. I skipped my game, calling in sick, and went home without talking to anyone. I closed my door and broke down in tears, feeling worthless.

For trying to respect this woman, I was cheated on. For giving my whole heart to this girl, I was cheated on. For being my authentic self with her, I was cheated on. I didn't know what to say, nor did I know how to process this pain. I was numb and felt used, played, and manipulated. I was reduced to a piece of meat. I felt dehumanized. I remember thinking, "Don't men do the cheating on women? I guess I'm not a man, am I?"

Why was I cheated on? I thought if I set the tone, she would've followed. Wasn't she a virgin too? What made her change? How could she say she was going to hold on to her virginity and wait for me too, but then sleep with another person she didn't even know? SHE WASN'T EVEN DRUNK! I gave my heart to this girl and really treated her with respect, and this was how she treated me back? I coughed so hard that I almost threw up. My spirit was crushed and my heart was broken. I could not believe that I had been cheated on. Was I not good enough? Maybe it was because I wasn't attractive and she was out of my league? Maybe I had to get bigger muscles?

This negative way of thinking didn't just last for a couple days. No, not even a couple weeks or months. It lasted for about a year. I was lifeless, fully dead, and couldn't get out of bed some days because my mind would just dwell on it.

Some of my friends heard what happened and they said, "Dude, you didn't smash? Anthony, you're an idiot. You had an opportunity to get laid. You're wasting your time and hers. Why didn't you have sex? Are you gay? Were you scared? Did you not know what to do? You know, you could've been one of the most popular kids if you'd slept with her! Come on, man. I'm trying to do you a favor. You're using your looks and personality to be made fun of instead of scoring women. I wish I had what you had; you're wasting your gifts. You know, it's still not too late to change people's opinions about you if you just hook up with her." The talk was relentless. All my friends and teammates were having sex and told me, "Don't be rude, bro. Girls have needs too. Show her you love her, man. Come on. She won't stay with you unless you have sex with her. Give her a reason to stay with you."

I began to blame myself and I questioned why I didn't sleep with her. Within a few hours, my dark thoughts turned into self-hatred.

I began to blame myself and I questioned why I didn't sleep with her. Within a few hours, my dark thoughts turned into self-hatred. This experience traumatized me and I began to resent holding on to my V-card. I saw it as a curse, not a blessing. I didn't even know why I'd chosen to wait at the time. All I could remember hearing was, "No sex. No. No.

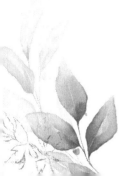

NO! Not until you're married." None of this blind obedience made any sense to me. What was so wrong with sleeping with someone before marriage when we loved each other? I began to stop caring what my inner circle told me. I felt they were manipulating my natural desire to have sex, and that they were old-fashioned and didn't know any better. I mean, it was 2015 at the time. I remember saying, "Who cares if I know a couple people who regretted their decisions in the past or have waited until marriage? I've seen better relationships than theirs."

All sorts of insecurities, questions, and doubts tormented my mind. I had many lonely late nights and early mornings full of despair, low self-esteem, lack of purpose, lack of passion, lack of identity, lack of love, and feelings of worthlessness. It was the beginning of my dark side. The beginning of doubting my worth and finding my value through the opinions of others. The beginning of losing my identity as Anthony John Simon.

You may be thinking the same thing I was back then and wondering *why* or *how* I chose to wait when I already *felt* in love? Maybe you had or have some questions about relationships, sex, love, and self-worth like I did. Before my stories and *whys* can actually make any sense to you, we need to be on the same page as to what sex actually is and isn't.

Well, I think it's about time I stop stalling and we finally talk about sex. Ohhhh, boy. Gentlemen, it's time to buckle up and put on your big-boy belts. Ladies, it's time to put on your big-girl pants. It's sex education time. WOOO, BABY!

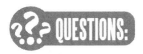

QUESTIONS:

1. Why do you think I didn't have sex with Katie?
2. Have you ever had an experience where you wouldn't compromise your standards but got hurt? Did you give up on your standards? Why or why not?
3. What are your insecurities, negative voice/self-talk, and fears or doubts when it comes to relationships?

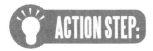

ACTION STEP:

1. Write down your very first heartbreak experience and how it shaped the way you view relationships. Feel free to share with me at coachanthonysimon@gmail.com

3

The Shameless Naked Truth About Sex

W e don't talk enough about sex.

"What? Anthony, all we see is sex. How can we not think about it when it's everywhere?"

Sure. Our culture is flooded with oceans' worth of information on sex. Computer screens, televisions, movies, radios, magazines, books, apps, websites, social media, and clubs all scream, "SEX SELLS!" Sex truly does sell, but who actually talks about sex—authentic, transcendent, pure sex? Instead, sex is twisted, perverted, cheapened, idolized, and used as a tool only for power, pleasure, filling one's insecurities, and covering up wounds and fears of rejection or even loneliness. It doesn't

Sex between two people who love each other body and soul is transcendent. More often than not, that's not the type of sex people are having.

take a smart person to see that people are slaves to toxic relationships they just can't get out of or are lowering their standards just so they can have glimpses of love, attention, or affirmation.

Sex is the strongest desire in our human nature. But desires need to be disciplined and under control in submission to our minds, otherwise we become slaves with selfish motives and impure hearts, living in lust instead of in love, and never reaching our fullest potential to be loved and to love fully.

Sex is pleasurable. Sex between two people who love each other body and soul is transcendent. More often than not, that's not the type of sex people are having.

If you're anything like me, you've been told that sex is bad, nothing special, or not supposed to be talked about. Parents, religious people, teachers, ministers, friends, or even famous speakers often refer you to the five S's: Suppressing, Socializing, Scolding, Shaming, and Scaring. These people always seem to box sex into the confines of dos and don'ts, rights and wrongs.

You'll understand when you hear these examples:

1. **Suppressing Sex:** "You're too young. Wait until you're married." "Don't think about sex or even say the word. Don't worry about that now." "Be quiet, I'm driving. I need to focus on my work. You're distracting me. Now's not the time."

2. **Socialized Sex:** "Sweetie, I don't want you turning wild in college, so I'd rather have you have sex in moderation than abnormally suppressing your desires and having you lose it and have sex with countless people. I mean sex is natural, after all, so you might as well be doing it." "I don't have to teach you about sex; just learn from the T.V., movies, or whatever the world says about it." As long as you're having sex with someone you love and you feel ready, it's okay with us. Just make sure to have safe sex and protect yourself." "Sex is normal. It's not that special. It's something you just do in the back of the movie theatres or outside to see if you're compatible with someone."

3. **Scolded Sex:** "SEX!! WHAT?!?! What did you say? Why are you using that word? Who taught you the word 'sex'? Where did you learn it from? BAD! WE DON'T USE THAT WORD IN THIS HOUSE! YOU KNOW BETTER!" "Tell me you're joking . . . you lost your virginity? I don't believe this. What

kind of a person are you? You're not good enough for anyone now. You might as well go sleep with anyone because you're a slut and nobody will take you. You already failed."

4. **Shamed Sex:** "It's just bad, so don't do it." "YOU SINNER! YOU'RE GOING TO HELL! HOW COULD YOU DO THAT? YOU SHOULD BE ASHAMED OF YOURSELF. YOU FAILURE. DID I NOT TELL YOU NO?!" "Your future spouse won't forgive you, nor will God." You're going to hell and it's too late."

5. **Scared Sex:** "You'll get a disease." "You'll get pregnant!" "You'll be a bad parent and your kids will get diseases if you don't." "You're going to suffer a lot. You don't see it now." "You'll never find true love if you do it because you'll live in regret the rest of your life." "You won't be able to forgive yourself and your spouse won't either. No sex before marriage because sex produces children and you aren't ready for that level of commitment. You aren't financially stable nor are you mature enough to handle the responsibilities that babies demand. So don't think about it now."

The problem is many people are subconsciously taught to perfect the negative perspective of sex: suppressing or sheltering you from receiving total free love, scolding the beauty and pleasure of sex, shaming sacred sex, scaring you into not having sex, or even reducing sex's true value to just a social, casual thing to do because the media says so. Viewing sex in these ways can lead to people feeling disconnected, upset, used, shameful, guilty, manipulated, or even abused under the sheets. This happens because nobody is addressing the aching, bleeding needs of your heart—informing you about the shameless naked truth about sex.

Viewing sex in these ways can lead to people feeling disconnected, upset, used, shameful, guilty, manipulated, or even abused under the sheets.

Why does our world have such mixed messages about sex? You've not only read about it right now, but you've also seen it. Some celebrate sex, some suppress it, some fear it, some glorify it, some shame it, and some think nothing of it but a thing to do when they're bored. Some can't decide how they feel about it.

What are your thoughts on sex? You've already got a message about sex resting in your conscious or unconscious mind. I'm serious, think about it right now. What do you think about sex? Be real with me and yourself because it's impossible for you to learn more truths about sex without knowing where you have already learned about it. You may have learned through home, movies, TV shows, porn, a shaming or silent church, an abusive relationship, a loved one who made you fear having sex with negative statistics, or even silent parents whose silence spoke louder than words. Think about it for a hot second . . . what experiences best described your sex education?

Why am I asking?

You may be believing a beautiful lie about sex, mistaking that lie for what sex actually is. I can sit here and tell you what I think about sex with credible, truthful information, statistics, and experiences in my life as well as the lives of others, but if you're already convinced you know what sex is and you think you have the best relationship, then you'll never receive a better love life. You've already made up your mind, not fully hearing what I have to say with an open mind and heart because you're hearing it through the filter of what you know or what you've experienced.

We've all learned something about sex, but most of us didn't receive a healthy foundation on what sex and love actually are, so our relationships suffer, both romantically and casually.

I want you to go back in time to the first time you learned about sex. Chances are, it wasn't one time, it was multiple times. When were those days and experiences? Reflect, reflect, reflect. You have to question the sources you learned from. Even question me. It's healthy to wrestle with everything because doubt will eventually lead you to the truth. We've all learned something about sex, but most of us didn't receive a healthy foundation on what sex and love actually are, so our relationships suffer, both romantically and casually.

Out of all these five main environments in which most of us learn about sex, the most common one is socializing sex. This is present in today's high schools, college campuses, and even middle schools.

SOCIALIZING SEX:

Sex sells. It couldn't be more true.

The culture around you is always talking about sex, through movies, jokes, casual conversations, relationships, TV shows, ads, and much, much more. Everything is accessible and nothing is hidden about sex. Your parents didn't need to talk to you about sex. Why would they? It was pressing all up in your face. Sex became a part of your life and you learned that it's okay to view sex as nothing more than a casual body-to-body physical experience—anything more is overthinking a casual hook-up to meet your needs and get the pleasure you want.

You may catch yourself saying, "Why do some people make such a big deal about sex? There's nothing sacred about it. I don't feel any 'soul tie' or spiritual/emotional connection when I have sex. Sex isn't a big deal; it's just a way of connecting on a physical level and showing my love to someone."

If you were raised viewing sex as casual, give me a chance in the next chapters to show you how your spirit, mind, soul, and body are exposed and vulnerable in sexual activity. You'll have a greater understanding of your worth, and the shining, liberating truths will bring a freedom to the dull, dark, beautiful lies about your current or previous relationships.

Unfortunately, many have grown deaf to these liberating truths and hear only the body saying, "Gimme pleasure. Me, me, me. It's all about me." No matter how numb you might be to the deepest parts of your soul and spirit, you can relate to the aching feelings of solitude and the desire for a greater intimacy to be seen and loved for who you truly are.

I'm going to be showing you the exact *whys* and *reasons,* but for now, just understand that this environment is a beautiful open room flooded with everything you've ever dreamed of. Once you enter, the door shuts, locks, and traps you inside until someone hears you screaming, "LET ME OUT!" and decides to break down the door and save you. Making sex an everyday experience and part of life may allow you to become more comfortable, but it will not give you the full truth about the right perspective of sex. You need wisdom, not only experience, to lead you to freedom, connection, unconditional love, and intimacy. You need the truth about sex, not just feelings about it.

Despite the media always talking about sex, they don't really talk about the authentic power, value, and the shameless naked truth about sex.

Despite the media always talking about sex, they don't really talk about the authentic power, value, and the shameless naked truth about sex. Your environment, upbringing, and culture has subconsciously taught you how to avoid diseases, infections, babies, committed relationships, and sacrifices when your nature really wants to know how to find, build, and maintain an intimate relationship of real love. This culture of death needs something that isn't just convincing or right to do, but rather something that addresses the deepest desires that your heart demands— to love and be loved at your fullest capacity.

Very few are taught to perfect the positive shameless naked truth about sex:

1. Expressing a powerful bonding love where two people come together and give their souls to each other as gifts, synchronizing and becoming one.
2. Delighting in shameless, pleasurable, beautiful, intimate sex that transcends any love you've ever received.

3. Understanding the freedom to have sex without pressure, guilt, or manipulation and being accepted for your authentic self.
4. Valuing and understanding the sacredness of sex, your worth, and standards.

Whenever I tell people who grew up in this culture about these life-hack secrets about sex, they always say, "I've never heard anything like it before. I can't believe I was being robbed all these years. How do I change?" This is because many people learned about sexuality in a negative religious/worldly manner focusing only on what is forbidden and what is allowed. Others learned about it through the lens of modern sex education, which reduces one's sexuality to biology and pleasure, disregarding the mental, emotional, and spiritual aspect of sex. This might count as 'sex ed,' but it's not a true education in human sexuality.

This leads us to the second environment—one that's just as common, especially among religious people.

SUPPRESSING, SCOLDING, SCARING AND SHAMING SEX:

When a list of rights and wrongs is all that's enforced, you begin to see intimacy and sex as a restricting, chaining rulebook instead of a liberating, free, romantic non-fiction book written inside your heart. But this love letter inside your heart explains all the *whys* to our questions and the *whats* should be framing and guiding our understanding of intimacy and sex.

Let me speak from my own personal experience here. I was always told the following in my environment:

"Sex? What is sex? I don't know what this 'sex' word is or means. Are you making up words?"

"Once you're married, you're going to have *THE BEST* experiences of your life. You'll have a sex slave who will do everything you desire and listen to whatever you tell them to do. Anything. Did you hear what I said? Anything. You're still too young now so don't even think about sex. Shame on you if you do, ya pervert. You're not married yet so don't worry about it. Just worry about holding on to your virginity and don't form relationships with women, otherwise you'll lose your virginity, get diseases, get a girl pregnant, and become heartbroken."

Uhhhhhh, yeah. . . . Welcome to my environment. This was my life growing up. In my community, nobody talked about the beauty of sex, and if they did mention it at all, it was only negative statistics, theology, or ideas. It was forbidden to talk about women in my environment, otherwise they'd think I was sleeping with a girl.

But this is unhealthy. Sex must be talked about.

Parents aren't talking about sex to their children, and if they are, they are usually uneducated on the topic, leaving their children more lost, confused, and restless than before because they're battling the natural desire to learn about sex. They feel like they're living a double life, knowing that they should be pure, but having thoughts and desires guided by their puberty. You can't blame them for being curious. Don't take it from my mouth, take it from others. Here, listen to these:

"The people in my life never told me anything about sex and I was left to figure it out on my own."

"I wish my parents had told me more about sex. I wouldn't have had to experience failed relationships. I could've saved so much time and heartache."

"Since my mom and dad didn't teach me about sex, I just watched movies, stayed up late at night watching TV, went on my iPhone, asked friends, looked at magazines, watched videos of people doing it, and read articles on sex."

"My parents didn't educate themselves on sex, so they would live in fear, be awkward, or make up lame answers that didn't meet the demands I had for wanting to know what sex was all about. Because they failed, I failed."

"I was always told, 'You'll learn about sex when you're older,' but I never did. Seemed like excuses to me. Now it's too late."

If the value of sex isn't being talked about in your environment, I don't blame you for going to the world to learn about sex and attempting to discover it on your own. That's what I did—I went to the world to understand and learn about sex. This caused a lot of problems that you'll find out about as you continue reading. Since I went through this journey of unveiling the mystery of sex on my own, I decided to go with whatever suited and sounded good to me for the moment. I fell into many traps and pits because I let the culture of death influence my perspective on sex instead of listening to informed, trusted voices. I learned about sex, sexuality, love, worth, and beauty from people who were just trying to make money off me—from pop culture. Society began to dictate what I should do with my body, what I should watch, and even what I should say in my relationships. These ideas became my beliefs and formed my perspective and identity on a counterfeit of love: lust.

> **I learned about sex, sexuality, love, worth, and beauty from people who were just trying to make money off me—from pop culture.**

There was a lot of resistance from my environment and I felt a lot of shame and even fear talking about sex—but the desire to talk about it was natural. I talked to a married couple who had a very similar experience to me. Listen to what they have to say.

"I always was told, 'Wait it out! Wait it out! Stay a virgin until you get married so you can give your full self to someone. Your wedding night will be this euphoric experience.' It worked. I miraculously was a virgin on my wedding night, but it was filled with unrealistic, false expectations of what sex would actually be like. I was disappointed and filled with pain because I still wasn't able to connect. I was confused, hurt, taken aback."

"I couldn't make the sudden change from hearing, 'Bad! Sex is bad and forbidden,' to 'Sex is good and permitted and natural.'"

Although this type of upbringing celebrates virginity during the wedding day, people still fail to understand the beauty and depth of sex. It's also a trap that leads to a dead end full of shame, regret, anger, and even insecurity.

So many people in this environment fall into the trap of thinking that virginity is the end-all, be-all. "I can't lose my virginity because I won't be accepted. I won't be worth much. Nobody will see my value. I can't be forgiven. I'm just trying to do what I've been told to do and hopefully I don't mess up." If you're living under this mentality, you're forcing yourself to be pure out of fear. You may also be saying, "How far is too far? How can I get away with the most possible and still call myself a virgin? Making out? Touching? Oral sex? Grinding? Hmmm."

You're saying, "I want to be pure because I need to be pure." I'm trying to get you to understand that being pure because you feel forced, guilt-tripped, or manipulated is not the right approach. Do it because you know the benefits of being pure. That's what this whole book is about. You must know why you want and need this in order to be healthy. Fear may be able to control your behavior, but it can't transform your heart and mind through your belief system.

Think relationship over rules, not rules over relationship. I don't want you to live under confining rules, never understanding the liberating truth, plan, and purpose about love. Hatred is not the opposite of love. Fear is. When you pursue any ideal outside of love, you will never produce love that remains.

Sex is a foreign language that requires time to study and learn. Sex isn't just an experience of pleasure.

Neither of these environments transfer to the reality of sex. Regardless of which background you might have grown up with about sex, know this for now: Sex is a foreign language that requires time to study and learn. Sex isn't just an experience of pleasure. Sex doesn't equal love if not done with proper timing, place, and position of heart.

If you feel ashamed of your past, or don't care about having a pure heart, keep reading. There's so much hope for you, as I'll be talking about in the next chapters. You can have a better relationship than so many people even with your past. In fact, it can actually be used for your good, but you must first learn exactly how much you're worth.

It's time for change. Change starts now. You're about to grow in wisdom and it's time to silence the silence of sex with the roaring truth about sex, love, and worth. I'm going to walk with you on this journey by informing and inspiring your mind and heart with the life-changing four-step process we talked about in the introduction of finding a transforming love:

1. Part I: Seeking Love and Worth—Mind and Heart Education
2. Part II: Finding Love and Worth—Mind and Heart Transformation
3. Part III: Building Love and Worth—Behavior Modification
4. Part IV: Giving Love and Worth—Sexual Liberation

Before you learn more about this four-step process, you must first learn how to free your mind to understand just how precious you are. It's time to stop guessing how much you're worth. Let's unlock this puzzle together.

Don't give up on me just yet, because I'm not giving up on you. This is the chapter you won't want to miss. I made sure to give it my all because I want your all. But I need you to do me a huge favor. Will you take my right hand so I can help lead you to the truth? Many run away from this journey. Will you be one of those many? There's only one way to find out. . . .

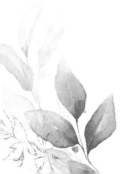

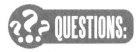

QUESTIONS:

1. What were you told about sex? Which environments did you grow up in? Write down everything you thought about it.
2. After reading this chapter, has your perspective on sex changed?
3. Why do you think purity of heart is more important than virginity?

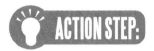

ACTION STEP:

1. Write down which sex environment you grew up in. Then, write down where you first learned about sex. Feel free to share them with me at coachanthonysimon@gmail.com

4

The Pearl Is Within You

Do you know where the wealthiest place in the world is?
China? Nope.

United States? Sorry, guess again.

Your toilet? Haha, good one.

Give up?

It's the graveyard.

"Anthony, what? The graveyard?" Yes, the graveyard. You'll find out why after reading this inspiring story.

Justin was a poor kid who was given a map by his uncle which said there was a pearl buried somewhere under his house. It took him three years to finally crack the secret message in the map and find out where the pearl was located. The map led him to a dark tunnel in the innermost depths of his house. Initially scared, Justin overcame his fear and went down the tunnel where he found a surprisingly shiny treasure chest. With the key he found using the map, he unlocked the treasure chest and found the shiniest pearl that mesmerized his eyes, leaving him speechless. Instead of taking the time to research how much the pearl was worth, he decided to save himself the hard work and bring it to a pearl specialist to tell him the value of the pearl. As Justin approached the pearl inspector, the inspector stared at Justin with a warm, welcoming look in his eyes.

Inspector: "Can I help you?"

Justin: "Hey! After three years of searching, I found this pearl. I'm sure it has some sort of value to it since it was hidden so well in a secret treasure chest."

Inspector: "Where did you find this pearl? Can you bring it closer so I can hold it?"

Justin: "Yeah, I found it buried in the depths of my house."

Inspector: "Let me see it. Oh, okay. I see. How much are you looking to get for this pearl? How much do you think it's worth?"

Justin: "I don't know; that's why I'm bringing it to you. I'm sure it's worth at least a couple thousand dollars. Right?"

Inspector: "Sorry, kid, you were scammed. Hate to break it to ya, but it's only worth a couple hundred. I can sell it for $100. I can't put it in the auction because it's not as valuable as you thought it would be. You sure you didn't get this thing at the dollar store and you're not tricking me? Look, I said I'll give you $100. That's more than enough, kid. Either you take the deal or you move out of the line and let the next person step forward."

Justin: "You're kidding me, right? Like, is the joke over already?"

Inspector: "NEXT! You heard me, I said, 'Next!' Is that not clear enough for you? Do you understand what 'next' means?"

Justin: "I worked my whole life for this pearl, man. You don't understand what I've been through. How many late nights I had losing my mind thinking I'd never find this pearl."

Inspector: "Look, we've got a line that's waiting; I don't have time for your emotions. This happens all the time. Stop making a scene, acting like you're more special than everyone else. Move on and accept the reality of the situation. I said I can take it for $100. At least you're getting something, man."

Justin decided $100 was better than having it sit on the shelf. He sold the pearl to the inspector and left the building. As he got in his car, he realized he'd left his car keys in the building. As he was going back inside the building to grab his keys, he was shocked to see that the same exact pearl he sold was being auctioned at $250,000. Within seconds, people were bidding and it ended up selling for $1,000,000.

Though heartbreaking, that's not the saddest part. Justin immediately yelled at the inspector saying, "Hey, you tricked me! That's my pearl. Give it back." The heartless, cold-blooded inspector was a complete jerk. He said, "A deal is a deal, kid. I gave you how much you valued the pearl for. You said a couple thousand and I brought it down to a hundred dollars for you. It's called wheeling and dealing. It's not my fault you didn't do your research on the pearl's value before you brought it in. Look, I'm a businessman and if you actually had a brain, you would've known businessmen don't care about your feelings. We just stir your feelings up and give you exactly how much you give yourself."

My heart goes out to Justin because he didn't even believe what he saw. He wondered how the pearl sold within seconds? Where did all the people just magically come from? I don't blame him for feeling torn apart, robbed, manipulated, used, cheated on, taken advantage of, and abused. How could he not have felt heartbroken? He had the prize in his hand, but because nobody instructed him on the value of pearls—what to look for and what not to look for—he was lost. Justin was torn as he sacrificed the pearl's truest value and worth by selling it for pennies.

I want you to put yourself in Justin's shoes. How would that make you feel? Imagine your whole life you went searching for this pearl, only to sell it for a couple bucks when it was worth a million dollars! What turned out to be real became fake in your eyes because somebody told you it wasn't worth anything. Doesn't it hurt that nobody taught you the value of the pearl? Nobody instructed you on what to look for and what not to look for. You could've found out on your own, but out of laziness, confusion, and lack of direction, you weren't able to take the necessary steps to discover the value of the pearl before it was too late.

UNLOCKING THE MYSTERY OF THE PEARL

The story you just read is an allegory. Justin is your ordinary human being who didn't have the discipline or guidance to find out the value of his pearl, so he got deceived by the inspector and manipulated into selling it for much less than its actual worth.

The pearl guarded by the treasure chest hidden in the house symbolizes your worth, which contains your whole self: physically, intellectually, mentally, emotionally, and spiritually. Put simply, the pearl is the total gift of your whole body and soul that you give to another person. Your sense of the value of your pearl increases as your understanding in love increases.

With proper mind and heart education, you can find your worth. And you do this by growing in the purity of your heart by seeking, finding, building, and giving unconditional love. How? Find your standards and live them out through your virtues. When you live out your standards through a proven virtue and value system, your mind and heart begin to transform. This leads to a pure heart, mind, and body, which leads to

When you live out your standards through a proven virtue and value system, your mind and heart begin to transform.

finding and giving pure love. Once you find authentic love, you build your worth by modifying your behavior and growing in the ability to love and be loved fully through the universal laws of love. Finally, you can experience sexual liberation by giving this love—your pearl—to someone who deserves it.

The pearl is the reward of eternal satisfaction you feel through living a life of purity in heart and growing in specific virtues known to grow love. Your ability to save your body is rewarding because it's an act of giving your entire self—physically, intellectually, mentally, emotionally, and spiritually—to a single person.

One cannot give what one does not possess. You must first possess the pearl by possessing the value of it. If you're not a master of self through purity of heart, you won't be capable of a lasting relationship.

Want to know the secret to finding a better relationship? Find your worth.

And how do you find your worth?

You must learn the universal loveable laws of love. You must also learn the specific virtues and standards that lead to unconditional love. It can't just be anything. You've got to have the right vision, otherwise without the correct vision, you'll drift away. Wanted love will turn into unwanted lust. The more you know yourself by encountering love, knowing love, and having a personal relationship with love, the more you can give yourself. You can't give what you don't already have. This is why so many people fail in their relationships. They think they know themselves, their dreams, their visions, and most importantly, they think they know love. But they don't. If they did, they wouldn't be in countless broken relationships. It's not their fault; they just don't understand the laws of love and how to live under them with the specific virtues.

So, what are the specific loveable laws of love and virtues that lead to encountering, knowing, and having a relationship with love? Think about it for a hot second.

Let's unlock the second mystery—the treasure chest.

UNLOCKING THE MYSTERY OF THE TREASURE CHEST

Although the pearl is precious and displays its worth through its outer beauty, it's nothing without its guardian—the treasure chest. The treasure chest represents your purity of heart, which gives you the ability to love and be loved the more you strengthen it with your virtues, values, and standards. If pearls aren't hidden and protected inside a sturdy treasure chest with a lock, they are worth nothing because they're easily accessible and easy to steal. So, to protect and value your worth, you must first learn to grow a pure heart and then guard your pearl (your worth) with your pure heart. Everything flows from a pure heart—your sex life, your worth, your identity, your purpose, and most importantly, your ability to love and be loved fully. The purer your heart, the more you're able to love and be loved at your fullest capacity.

Virginity is a fruit that grows from the tree called purity of heart. Purity of heart has more weight than virginity does.

If you thought the treasure chest represented your virginity, guess again. Virginity is great, but truly it isn't the end-all, be-all. More on this later. What matters is having a pure heart—a heart that understands the truth about what it means to be fully seen and what it means to love and be loved at your fullest capacity. Virginity is a fruit that grows from the tree called purity of heart. Purity of heart has more weight than virginity does. Since purity should come before virginity, it has a higher price and makes up your full worth. To prove my point, there are a lot of marriages who had slept with multiple people before marrying their spouse and they have some of the strongest marriages I've ever seen. How? More on this later, but know they've experienced deep forgiveness and mercy. One way to experience deep love is through being on the opposite end . . . deep lust. How can you appreciate the good days if you've never felt the bad days?

So, what exactly is purity of heart? For now, know that purity of heart is the power which frees love from selfishness, aggression, fear, bitterness, or wounds. To the degree that a person weakens their

31

purity of heart, his or her love becomes more and more selfish, that is, satisfying a desire for selfish pleasure and no longer selfless love.

The trick is to discover how pure your heart can actually be. How much can you grow in the purity of your heart to master yourself and give your full self to someone who deserves it?

UNLOCKING THE MYSTERY OF THE HOUSE

Your house symbolizes your standards, yet another guardian to the greatest treasure: your worth. Your standards create and protect the vision of your worth you require of yourself and others by the virtues and values you live out according to the universal truths and principles of love.

Not everyone can come into your house, and every house has different standards (rules) of who's allowed and who isn't. These are the people you allow into your life—your inner circle. Those who enter are a part of your inner circle; they bring significance to your life and should have the same standards as you do. When someone comes to your house, if they annoy you, manipulate you, upset you, belittle you, threaten you, or even break things, you kick them out without any doubts or hesitation. Anyone who doesn't have your standards should be kicked out of your life because they aren't bringing you up, they're bringing you down. You've got to set boundaries, which are the rules that are guided by your virtues and values.

Even if someone were to come to your house, you must learn to build trust to show that person your treasure chest and most prized possession. You don't just cast your pearls to swine just so they can spit them back at you sloppy, wet, and chipped to many pieces with no more value. What I'm saying is, you don't just give anyone the map to find your pearl and the key to your treasure chest. You give it to only one person who you deeply trust. Even if someone earned your trust and you showed them where the treasure chest is (your pure heart, aka your true personality), you wouldn't give them your most valuable possession

Sex, Love & Worth

for nothing. You'd expect them to bring their pearl, too. The gift of your pearl needs to be guarded from whatever—or whoever—might degrade it.

UNLOCKING THE MYSTERY OF THE INSPECTOR AND BUYER:

The pearl inspector represents the evil leaders of our culture and false relationships whose only job is to kill, steal, rob, and decrease the worth of other people to increase their money and selfish, impure hearts by manipulating your uninformed, pure heart. They only care to get rich, or to get pleasure from seeing you suffer because they can't get over the same bitter past Justin went through. Out of laziness and lack of guidance to seek the truth about the pearl's value, Justin failed to do the research himself and just went to the inspector to find out the value. Similarly, in our world, we lack knowledge on our worth because our environment failed to teach us, so we go with the flow by trusting others and listening to the world's opinions and affirmations about our worth. Instead of telling the world how much we're worth, we let the world tell us. Justin selling the pearl to the inspector reaffirms that the competition is real. The $100 he received represents the amount of love you received based on the knowledge of love you had and the amount of virtue you had.

The inspector took advantage of Justin. But he had buyers who were willing to pay the true price for the pearl. You've got to find the right buyer who knows how much you're worth. Someone who's willing to buy your pearl at full price because they would never sell their pearl for even 99.999 percent of the value they know it's worth. There are always buyers out there who are willing to not only pay your full price but more. That's why the pearl was auctioned for what it was worth—$250,000— but it sold for more—$1,000,000.

The buyer who pays full price for it understands the journey you took to get there, which symbolizes the greater meaning of love.

Love isn't love until it has cost you something to give it away: sacrifice through self-denial, discipline, controlling your emotions, surrender, servanthood, stepping into your fears and facing them, going against the current, and holding firm to your vision through persistence and consistency.

Don't market your pearl at 50 percent out of desperation, hoping it will sell because you're seemingly broke. Have hope. You want someone who is willing to offer you more than your full value because you're one of a kind.

> **You want someone who is willing to offer you more than your full value because you're one of a kind.**

Do you now see how the graveyard is the wealthiest place in the world? Many of us die never finding our identity and realizing our worth. It's sad to say, but our dreams of finding love die with us in the graveyard, and dreams are the richest forms of currency.

I don't want you to die never realizing your fullest potential. I don't want you to die never knowing you were made for more love. Please. You've got to understand that I'm going to do everything in my power begging you to wake up and change.

When you don't know just how precious and valuable you are, you allow others to put a price tag on you, market you, and sell you for waayyyy less than what you're actually worth. You may be searching for your worth in others because you don't know where to find your worth . . . but that's going to change this chapter. I'm going to walk you step by step, dude. I'm going to teach you how to draw living water from your empty, broken water bucket.

You can't fake your worth. People can sense that, and that's why you may be manipulated, laughed at, or even taken advantage of. You either know it or you don't. If you don't know it, the world will tell you what you're worth, just like the inspector told the man. It's not enough to just believe you're as valuable as a million-dollar pearl. You must *know* it. How do you know it? By living it out.

The question is, how do you know? How do you truly know what your actual worth is? For starters, it's important to note that your worth comes from the degree of how pure your heart is. The purer your heart, the more you're able to love and be loved. How much love can you actually receive in your cup and pour onto others, though? Are you worth 128 ounces of love? What about sixty-four ounces? Maybe eight ounces?

Not getting it?

Everyone is born with a different amount of love they can receive and give. That's what makes us human. We all have different gifts, talents, and charisms we can use to love and be loved differently, which is why we all have different amounts of love we can receive and give.

Imagine you have a cup that holds 128 ounces, while someone else to your left and right have empty cups at eight and sixty-four ounces, respectively. Your job isn't to listen to others telling you that you're only worth eight ounces of love when you know that's not right. Your job is to not only fill your cup with 128 ounces of love, but to also strive to have it overflow so that others can fill their cups through yours.

This is the greatest secret there is to love and finding love. Learn to overflow your cup with so much love that others who are empty or even full will naturally be attracted to you.

UNLOCKING THE MYSTERY OF THE MAP AND KEY

Many of us are handed a map, just like Justin was, that leads us to unlocking and finding our worth, but out of laziness, fear, doubt, lack of patience, lack of trust, or even carelessness we decide to quit or give up. Heck, even ignorance or lack of guidance causes us to not want to date ourselves because we don't even know what to do or where to start, so we allow the world to tell us. Although Justin passed the first test, he didn't close strong by finding out just how special his pearl was. The map represents the specific virtues that lead you to finding the key to the loveable laws of love to unlock a pure heart, which leads to understanding of our worth.

Some of us find the key to unlocking the treasure chest that holds our worth but we don't do the research to find out how much we are worth. The research in this case represents dating ourselves by building ourselves through these universal standards, virtues, and values to be loved and to love at our fullest capacity. Date yourself. Take yourself out for a steak dinner and wine and get to know you. (Seriously! I'll cover this in the next chapter.)

Learn to date yourself and grow in specific virtues, values, and standards that I will be mentioning in the next chapters. When you can date yourself, you start to have a personal relationship with love and you begin to understand what love is and isn't. When I say date yourself, I'm asking you to ask yourself the hard questions that nobody thinks about anymore:

1. What do you want in a relationship? What are the non-negotiable needs you require in someone? These are your standards.
2. Who are you? How do you know what is true about you and what isn't? Why are you here on planet Earth? What's your purpose in life? What were you created to do? Why does your life have meaning?
3. What forms your identity? What do you value the most in life? What's your vision? Deepest dreams? Can you create deeper dreams? Is there another dimension or level to these dreams?
4. What does your heart and mind tell you you're worth? What's the limit? Is there a limit? How do you find out the limit?
5. How do you find the truth about these universal laws of love that reveal what love is and isn't?
6. How do you grow in the ability to love and be loved? How do you love and be loved at your fullest capacity? How do you find unconditional love to reveal your passions, purpose, and meaning in life?

7. How much love does your heart want? Are you even worthy of getting that much love? How do you understand more about love? How much love do you desire?

The deeper you can answer these questions, the deeper your worth becomes. In other words, the more research you do, the greater love you receive and give through the standards you live out for yourself and require in others.

So, you know you need a vision, virtue, and value system, and the principles love demands, but how do you find that? This is what I meant by doing the research—finding your worth by fulfilling the flourishing vision of your worth and who you actually are instead of having others (the inspector) create a diminishing, false vision of your worth and who you are.

> **The deeper you can answer these questions, the deeper your worth becomes.**

How do you answer these questions? How do you do your "research," so to speak? How do you know what your standards are? How high is too high? What's realistic? How do you find a vision? How do you know which virtues to harness? What are the loveable laws of love? What's not a beautiful lie in disguise as the truth? These are good questions.

Is there a proven value and virtue system that works? Are there universal truths to creating a vision that leads to meeting love face-to-face, eye-to-eye, and heart-to-heart? Hmmmmmmm. What do you think? (These are secrets for the next chapters. Come on, I've gotta make this book somewhat entertaining and interactive. Don't get mad at me yet—you'll thank me later!)

When you're done, let me know what you came up with, and I'll see you soon. I gotta go see my lover; it's 3:03 p.m. right now and I promised I'd be somewhere in thirty minutes. (Oooof, I hope I make it in time. It's hard living two lives, but so worth it, haha.)

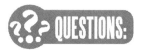

QUESTIONS:

1. Have you ever thought about how precious you are? Who in your life have you allowed to define how much you're worth?
2. How do you think you can increase your worth? Do you find yourself acting a bit like Justin? Is there any research you could be doing to help you determine your true worth? Do you know who you are?
3. What are your standards? Have you answered all the questions I asked you in this chapter? Write down your answers to all of them, or at least think about them carefully.

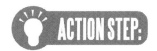

ACTION STEP:

1. Write down your answers to the seven questions listed above. Feel free to share them with me at coachanthonysimon@gmail.com

5

Creating the Vision in the Love Lab

When I was a part of my basketball team in college, our team had a vision of winning a section championship and entering into the March Madness tournament. Some of the players connected with this vision so deeply that they imagined that they already had the trophy in their hands.

To bring this vision into a reality, our team set high standards choosing to discipline and control unpredictable emotions. Collectively, our team was determined to grow in virtue through specific habits and rituals, which required sacrifice through self-denial, discipline, surrender, servanthood, stepping into fears and facing them, going against the current, and holding firm to the vision through persistence and consistency. Many hours were logged in whether that was getting shots up late at night, early morning workouts in the weight room, film, or eating recommended healthy foods that would maximize muscle growth and recovery.

What's crazy is what was once visualized actually ended up becoming a reality. Our team won the section championship finals game, allowing us to enter the March Madness tournament.

As a team, we received a trophy that symbolized our story of heroism and sacrifice. You have to understand something: this wasn't just any trophy for winning any game, nor was it a participation trophy. This was a section championship trophy. All the conference games added up to this one moment, and we did it. We won. We were actually holding the trophy in our hands.

This is the power of having a vision. You're able to step into the future and manifest it into a reality.

This only happened because we stepped into the future and made a deep emotional connection, feeling what it would feel like to receive the trophy. This is the power of having a vision. You're able to step into the future and manifest it into a reality.

All human beings desire unconditional love, unconditional truth, unconditional goodness (justice), unconditional beauty, and unconditional happiness (home). You must create an accurate vision of how you're going to get there. Without a specific and measurable vision, you won't ever find any of these five desires every human being longs for. I need you to make a decision: decide who you're going to be, why you're going to be that, and how you're going to become that. Make a decision about how you're going to get these five desires fulfilled.

Where there is no vision, you will perish and die because you end up spending all of your energy either trying to find pleasure or working to stay out of pain.

Where there is no vision, you will perish and die because you end up spending all of your energy either trying to find pleasure or working to stay out of pain. You must learn to stand for something, otherwise you stand for nothing and people will stand on you. If you have no standards, virtues, principles, or values, you will be walked all over, manipulated, used, abused, and confused.

Most of the people in the world never get taught how to keep their vision or dreams for these five desires alive. They may feel they need change, but they're just lost and don't know what to do. This is why many relationships fail: It's due to a lack of information and inspiration to change. Some have the vision, but they lower their standards and compromise and complain that they aren't meeting any of these five desires. Are any of these you? Are you lost, compromising, or lowering your standards in hopes of fulfilling these five desires in another person?

There is a formula for turning a relationship into a reality, but it takes self-control, courage, patience, persistence, wisdom, integrity, and humility. You need to write an emotional, sensory-rich statement of what your love life is going to feel like, look like, smell like, taste like, and sound like when you receive your relationship. The more emotional you make the statement, the more real it becomes. As you review this statement, you'll make it more and more clear and more and more powerful each time you write it and rewrite it and rewrite it again. You will find yourself living into this vision of unconditional love that you have described on paper if you live out this equation.

CREATING THE VISION (SETTING STANDARDS, VIRTUES, AND VALUES)

What are your love life and relationship going to look like, smell like, sound like, and feel like? How will they support, protect, or provide for you? How will they comfort, serve, or encourage you?

Remember, I asked you if there was a secret standard that was actually set? The equation? Well, guess what—there is one! There are universal, specific virtues that'll lead you to finding the loveable laws of love so you can encounter, know, and have a relationship with unconditional love. I'm saving you a ton of research by revealing these to you. You will find out the loveable laws of love, which will tell you how much you're worth, if you cultivate these virtues:

1. **Humility:** Striving to know yourself and unlock your fullest worth by being real despite the pain. Seeing yourself as you are and understanding you don't know it all.

2. **Wisdom:** Informing and inspiring your mind and heart about the universal truths of love and your worth, and how to apply them to relationships.

3. **Self-Control:** Being able to discipline your emotions through patience, self-denial (delayed gratification), and controlling your feelings (desires) with facts. Being able to manage yourself without external circumstances dictating your needs.

4. **Courage:** Deciding to never give up on your vision and do whatever it takes to get there despite having fears and doubts. Confronting your weaknesses and past despite the pain and comfort required to do so.

5. **Integrity:** Living out these virtues and holding firm to your vision despite the opinions, attention, or affirmations from others you do or don't get.

> **Virtues on the road to achievement cannot be achieved without disciplined and consistent habits and rituals.**

Visions without virtues are just visions that ultimately fuel disappointment. Virtues on the road to achievement cannot be achieved without disciplined and consistent habits and rituals.

As a certified personal trainer, I always tell my clients that in order to become a healthy person, you must first think like a healthy person. Once you begin to identify how your mind differs from someone who has the results you have, you'll begin to know how to take action. Most of us fail because we don't know how to take action. It's one thing to perish because we have no vision, but it's another to perish because we have a vision but don't know how to execute and bring that dream into fruition.

If you're trying to lose weight yet you're still overeating because you're lonely, anxious, depressed, heartbroken, or even bored, you still don't have the mind of a healthy person. You must first continue to discipline yourself with the intellect (mind) of a healthy person so your passions (emotions) and flesh don't dictate your decisions. You must learn to delay gratification and get greater control over your behavior, so that you can break the patterns that keep sabotaging you.

For some of you, you're consciously having sex with others hoping to find love, connect with someone, and meet these five non-negotiable needs of your soul. You have the vision to find unconditional love, but you're not finding it because you keep giving yourself away before finding yourself. You begin to decrease in the virtues I mentioned above, which only decreases your worth.

This is why you have so many off-days in your current relationship where you don't feel loved, seen, or even understood. This is also why you can't seem to find meaning, purpose, courage, or even what you're passionate about in life. You convince yourself, saying, "It's just a rough day," or "Yeah, I guess this job is all right." Or perhaps you're saying, "I'll find what I love to do one day. These wounds will just disappear on their own if I shove them deep down." Life was never supposed to be a *rough* day or only *all right* or even living under a past that burdens you. You're not supposed to just be satisfied—you're supposed to have life abundantly, being fully alive.

Let me explain. As you decrease in patience, selflessness, discipline, self-control, integrity, courage, humility, sacrifice, wisdom, compassion, and love through the purity of your heart, you lose your mind and become a slave to never truly understanding your worth because you never find and grow in the loveable laws of love. When you lose your mind, you lose your ability to recognize what it means to love and be loved at your fullest capacity. When you lose your ability to be loved and love at your fullest capacity, you lose the purity of your heart, which makes you lose your vision, standards, and values. When you lose these things, you lose your identity, worth, and meaning in life.

> **Every person seeks to be affirmed in his or her full value, which fulfills the deepest desire of the human heart: to see and be seen in full love.**

Every person seeks to be affirmed in his

43

or her full value, which fulfills the deepest desire of the human heart: to see and be seen in full love. Patience, selflessness through sacrifice, self-control, wisdom, humility, discipline, and an understanding of love and your worth enables everyone to be a gift received, not an object to be grasped. So, how do you become a gift to be received and not an object to be grasped? It's finally time. Let's check out the loveable laws of love and you'll see exactly what I mean.

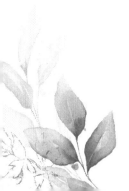

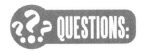 **QUESTIONS:**

1. Have you ever had a vision of what love is? What happened to that vision? Is it still alive? Why or why not?
2. What does having a pure heart mean to you? Is that a feeling or an actual fact? How can you tell?
3. What virtues do you need to work on to continue holding firm to your vision? How can you develop them?

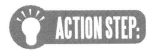 **ACTION STEP:**

1. Write out all 5 virtues mentioned in this chapter. Now, write a way to grow in each virtue and get to work. Feel free to message me your thoughts at <u>coachanthonysimon@gmail.com</u>

6

The Loveable Laws of Love

I want to be loved. You want to be loved. Even your greatest enemy wants to be loved. But it's not enough to desire love—you must work for it under the laws that love demands. We all desire to be loved, but how do you get into that relationship, stay in it, or get out of it ASAP? Are you really in a relationship of love, or is it lust? How do you know you're not just being used? Can you really trust their words, or are you unwittingly being led down a road paved to hell disguised as heaven?

Love is a good thing, but even a good thing can become destructive if it's used in the wrong way. Intention isn't enough. You must abide by the laws that love operates on. First, you must understand that the value of a relationship isn't defined by the intensity of the feelings, because feelings are like wind and rain: they come and go.

Most relationships end on a sour note because they promise love but give lust, which leads us to feel more insecure, bitter, and worthless than when we started.

Most relationships end on a sour note because they promise love but give lust, which leads us to feel more insecure, bitter, and worthless than when we started. I was debating about sharing my previous story with you since it's so candid and embarrassing, but knew I had to because so many of us are going through very similar experiences. So, how do you know when you love someone the right way?

Many of us confuse emotions with love. We live our life based on how we feel, which isn't always a bad thing, but you will be riding a

If you don't discipline your emotions, they will discipline you.

never-ending roller coaster that makes you nauseous and you'll eventually throw up all over your boyfriend or girlfriend. You have to be able to control your emotions—your passions—with your mind—your intellect. If you don't discipline your emotions, they will discipline you.

Now are you starting to see why it's essential to put love to the test with the loveable laws of love? If you don't, your emotions will lead you astray. You have to view the scenario from a non-judgmental, biased perspective by taming your feelings with logic. You see, you've got to understand that you may feel like you're "in love," but emotions don't create a lasting relationship; rather, what does is making the conscious decision to stay together no matter what emotion comes or goes. That's a part of true love: sacrifice.

TRUE LOVE STORIES

So, what are the loveable laws of love? Before I give you the answers, listen to what these couples in successful marriages who understand true love have to say:

"I never knew marrying my best friend would be this fun. Every day I feel like I'm dreaming, and it only gets better."

"The world says marry someone you could live with. I didn't do that. I married someone I couldn't live without. Without my wife, I would never be this happy. I'm a lucky ugly man. Don't know what she saw in me, haha!"

"The saying 'You only fall in love once' isn't true. Every time I look at my husband, I fall in love all over again. I'm so glad he loves me with all his heart, mind, body, and soul."

"I love being married. It's so great to find one special person you want to annoy for the rest of your life. I don't have to worry about being someone I'm not. She accepts me for my goofiness."

"'Since my husband decided to wait until marriage to have sex with me, it showed me he was serious about pursuing me. He was very creative with showing his love for me. This built our relationship in every aspect."

"The best love is the kind that awakens the soul. A love that makes both of us reach for more. This love is a fire in our hearts that brings peace to our minds knowing we have the same vision . . . That's what we hope to give each other forever."

Want a relationship like theirs?

Dudes. That's inspiring. So inspiring it led me to believe that unconditional love truly is possible. They each shared the same universal principles that made their relationships skyrocket to another dimension. How? They knew the four types of love that make any relationship flourish.

THE FOUR TYPES OF LOVE

Everyone claims to know what love is, but do they really, or are you just another dollar sign or toy being used and tossed aside when bored? So many people confuse love with lust at every angle. Many of us search for the meaning of love in poems, novels, books, films, songs, and videos, and we test relationship after relationship only to become more heartbroken and restless. Some believe love is found in purity while others believe the belief that love is lust of no fault of their own. Where

If you can't receive love, you can't give it out because you can't give what you don't already have.

do you stand? If you don't stand for anything, you stand for nothing. Do you stand for love or lust? What do you want? If you don't consciously program your mind for love, it will naturally program for lust.

You must first learn to inform your mind

and heart about what love is and isn't, otherwise you can never position yourself to receive love. If you can't receive love, you can't give it out because you can't give what you don't already have.

If you don't, you'll fall victim to the traps of the world and become programmed. Once again, if you don't stand for anything, you stand for nothing. In other words, if you don't program your mind, someone else will program it for you with beautiful lies.

For now, I want you to delete everything society has painted love to be in your mind. Imagine you have a bookshelf filled with books on love. Throw them all to the ground for now. You can re-add anything truthful after seeing this list.

Are you ready to finally find the map and key, and enter the coordinates in your mind to find selfless, pure love?

Let's start.

Yes, sex leads to one aspect of love, but it isn't the only one. Many think sex equals love, but it is only one aspect of love. The Greeks represented love with four words, while the English language only uses one. Many of the greatest psychologists, scholars, philosophers, church leaders, and successful marriages agree that these four loveable laws of love are what make a flourishing relationship.

These are the four loveable laws of love:

1. **Storge:** A familiar, affectionate bond that develops naturally with people or things that surround you. Think of family members, best friends, or people you see on the daily.
2. **Philia:** A powerful emotional bond in deep relationships that includes care, respect, and compassion for people who are compatible and share the same values. Think of your frat bros or sororities. They are closely knitted together as brothers and sisters by choice, not blood.
3. **Eros:** A passion or desire not only of a sexual nature, but also of an aesthetic or spiritual nature for what is considered beautiful and desirable. It's also defined as a passion that is sensual or

romantic including sexual desire, physical attraction, and physical love. Think sex.

4. **Agape:** Agape is the highest form of love. All three loves—storge, philia, and eros—flow from agape. Agape is unconditional, sacrificial, pure, selfless, forgiving love that wills the good of another by self-giving without seeking any reward or pleasure in return. This love is the most important of the three other loves. Think the greatest pure love you've ever received. Think the greatest good.

For your relationships and love to be authentic and successful like the quotes you read above, you need to have all four types of love—the loveable loves. No relationship can survive even with three of these loves. Because people don't know about these hidden loves, or they refuse to practice them, they suffer the consequences of broken hearts, failed relationships, or even divorce.

What you win a person with is what you keep them with.

What you win a person with is what you keep them with. If the other person is won over by the allure of pleasure, then the relationship will fade. After all, pleasure is repeatable; it can be obtained from any number of sources. However, the human person is unrepeatable. If you win a person with who you are, this gift cannot be repeated or replaced.

Imagine a three-legged chair. If one of the legs comes off, the whole chair collapses. It's the same with your current or future relationships. So many people only live or start their relationship in the eros love (sex),

Without the other three loves, your relationship will always fail, no matter who you are or what you say.

and it turns into lust because they haven't experienced the rest of the loves. They base their foundation on sex and wonder why they can't connect intellectually, mentally, emotionally, or spiritually. This leads to a break-up because they find someone more attractive or who is better in the bedroom.

You cannot just start a relationship with sex. Sex is the engine that gets the car to drive, but you need the rest of the parts: the wheels, the seats, the transmission, etc. Without the other three loves, your relationship will always fail, no matter who you are or what you say. There's always someone hotter or better. Your standard cannot be sex. Sure, I get it, you're the one exception reading this. You're different than everyone else. All right, cool, my dude. You may be sticking your relationship out, but failing doesn't always mean relationships ending; failing also means not getting your needs met. Failing also means not living life fully alive. Failing means you're in a toxic relationship. Failing means you're not being seen or loved as you ought to be. Failing means you're not living up to your full worth when you think you are.

Guys. Gals. There's another dimension of love you could be experiencing. Not even another level, another dimension, but you must first learn how to develop the other loves. Remember, to develop these loves, you must learn how to grow in the purity of your heart. This comes by growing in humility, wisdom, self-control, patience, courage, and integrity.

WHAT DOES UNCONDITIONAL LOVE (AGAPE) LOOK LIKE?

"Anthony, if I get all the three loves from agape, how do I get it? I want an example of unconditional love."

All right, my dawg. I gotcha. Hold on, let me think of one for a second. Okay, I got it. Unconditional love is when a puppy licks your face.

How is that relevant? It's not. I hope that made you laugh and smile. Dude, seriously? All right fine, unconditional love is when a puppy licks your face . . . even after you left the puppy alone all day in its cage. Unconditional love is about wanting the other person to be happy, no matter what. This is what we can learn from puppies.

True unconditional love is possible. The world programs your mind to think conditional love is the only form of love. You hear it when people say with their words and actions, "I love you if you are the way I want you to be." If you want to learn agape, unconditional love, you've got to have a deep relationship with love itself first. More on this later, but for now, let's go over the basics.

Unconditional love means accepting others despite their weaknesses, flaws, imperfections, or quirks.

Unconditional love knows no bounds. Unconditional love means accepting others despite their weaknesses, flaws, imperfections, or quirks. Unconditional love means showing mercy and forgiveness to others time and time again. Agape believes in all, cares for all, transforms all, and most importantly, strengthens and saves all. Agape never gives up on others and will chase you like a dog chasing a car.

"What's up with the dogs, dawg?" I don't know, dawg, I just love dogs, dawg. But seriously, even though you may drive thirty-three miles away from your house, the dog will keep chasing you. Even though the dog may have no more energy, be tired, or feel hurt or neglected, the dog stays hopeful that you may stop at a stop sign or stop light so it can potentially grab your attention for a split second. The dog will keep barking even though you are blasting your music until it captures even an ounce of your heart by getting in front of your car and forcing you to stop, otherwise you'll run your dog over.

Unconditional love means you care for another person's happiness more than your own, no matter how painful the choices you face may be. Think of someone dying for your life. Think of laying one's life down for another. After many years of failing, mistakes, and heartbreaks, I finally understood that love is not what you say, but love is what you do. Love is not a feeling, love is a choice. It's an action. The puppy still chooses to love even when it's locked in its cage all day with unmet needs. The dog still chooses to love by chasing you thirty-three miles away from your house.

True love is knowing a person's faults and loving them even more for them, not leaving them even sooner.

True, pure love is a journey with storms that will eventually clear out with beauty brought about. True love is knowing a person's faults and loving them even more for them, not leaving them even sooner. Love does not mean you will always agree, feel good, see eye-to-eye, or never have problematic arguments; it means despite the bad days with empty feelings, you still can't see yourself without that person.

If you want to receive unconditional love, you must give unconditional love. You must give what you want to receive. If you want more love, you must be more loving. If you want to be known and respected for your true worth, you must learn to give others the respect of their true worth. Don't be the guy or gal who gives just to receive. A pure heart gives without expecting anything in return—you must do the same. If you don't, everyone will know your love is fake and it won't last.

Remember the pearl?

I can't give you my pearl worth a million dollars if I don't own the pearl *yet*. I can sit you down with some wine, lean steak with broccoli, and romantic music, persuading you with empty promises and beautiful lies, saying, "I'll give you the pearl after we finish dinner." If you believe I have the pearl but you haven't even seen it yet, you're being played. I'll tell you, "I'll give you the pearl, but first give me the money." I'll try and persuade you to give me the money first, saying I have the pearl coming in a couple days and will give it to you then.

The same goes for love. You have to learn when someone is bluffing or not. That's what I'm going to teach you in this book. I'll teach you how to know if you're in a relationship of love or lust. Finding a relationship of love isn't always as clear as it may seem, which is why you may have some secret frustrations in your relationship you've suppressed. Lust is present when all four loves aren't present.

Most people out there are wolves in sheep's clothing. They may even show you a fake pearl, tricking you into believing it's real. You have to carefully study and examine every pearl because you can't afford to lose all the money you've worked hard for.

You could also be in the opposite side. You may think you've received a real pearl only to find out it was a fake pearl when it rained on your pearl one day. Then you realized it was spray-painted and had lost its beauty; the paint made it appear shiny on the outside but it was hollow on the inside all along. You may have been convinced in the moment because your emotions were played with, so you sold your pearl to get your money's worth. As the inspector looked at your pearl, he said, "Sorry, that's not an authentic pearl. It's a decoy; it's only worth pennies. Although it appears to be shiny on the outside, it's hollow on the inside."

> *It's not enough to just think your relationship is based on love— you must know.*

This is why so many relationships I got into failed. I didn't understand these four universal laws of love, and neither did the people I dated. Our relationships were based on lust and not love. It's not enough to just think your relationship is based on love—you must know. Everyone thinks they're in love, but if that were true, why do so many relationships fail? I know you and I aren't the only ones who have suffered and endured a form of rejection.

LOVE IS A CHOICE:

We often think of love as an emotion or an experience. Maybe it's the warm, electrifying pleasure you feel in a relationship, the physical and emotional desire to be close to another. While the emotional aspect of love is pleasurable, warm, intimate, close, exciting, electrifying, and transcendent, if you limit your understanding of love to the experiences of eros, you'll never have a solid, stable foundation of love. Love is built on choices, not feelings. Feelings don't last, choices do. That's why unconditional love is a choice. It's not dependent upon feelings or changing circumstances. Unconditional love endures under any trial, test, or circumstance.

> *Love is built on choices, not feelings. Feelings don't last, choices do.*

True love is honesty and trust. Love is mutual respect. Love is helping one another. Love is reaching your dreams together. Love is the connection of two hearts and minds. Love is selflessly helping one another. Love is taking a risk.

Love is an unconditional commitment to an imperfect person. Love is giving someone the power to destroy you, yet trusting them not to. To love somebody isn't just a strong feeling. It is a decision. Love is a promise. Love is a choice. A choice to be gentle. A choice to be patient. A choice to trust someone wholeheartedly. A choice to treat others with respect. A choice to listen to the spoken and unspoken words of others. A choice to treat others with mercy despite anger. Love is a choice to be selfless.

Love fixes everything. Love heals everything. Love forgives everything. Love transforms everything. Love produces everything. Love is everything.

Love between man and woman cannot be built without sacrifices and ordering your sexual desires to selflessness instead of selfishness. You will not be satisfied with anything less. You have everything to gain if you grow in these virtues and nothing to lose.

In an age in which people expect instant gratification, pleasure, and selfishness, patience and self-control over sexual desires to test your love proclaims a challenge of sacrifice and redirecting your sexual desire to get to know the person. Know that this purity of mind, heart, and body is possible. As a twenty-two-year-old virgin who found his lover, I know it's possible—and well worth it.

Love is a gift of self, not a gift to self. You have to learn how to control your impatient desire for oneness with patience, otherwise you will be dependent on pleasure in order to feel close and, before you know it, your relationship is only based on sex, which will rob you of the opportunity to be fully committed to each other.

Love is a gift of self, not a gift to self. If you can't conquer your lust, how can you ever love your spouse? You'll only use your spouse for your own sexual pleasure, which is lust. You can't give something if you're still a slave to something else.

When it comes to love, there is no place for selfishness, fear, insecurity, doubt, or lack of trust. When love makes demands, don't back down, but accept the challenge. True love begins when nothing is looked for in return. For love to be real, you must empty yourself and your desires first and fill yourself with your lover. Do not accept as love a relationship which lacks Agape! If someone says they love you, but their actions demonstrate otherwise because they haven't taken the time to get to know you emotionally and spiritually, then they're lying. Do not accept any love that lacks truth. This is why you must have purity of heart.

WHAT EXACTLY IS PURITY OF HEART?

Purity of heart is taking this definition of love to will the good of another by helping them become the best version of themselves and fulfill their truest potential, and applying that to sex. A good sex life involves purity of heart by practicing patience and controlling your sexual desires and thoughts by gaining discipline over your body. Purity of heart is understanding the value of sex, seeing it as a gift, and growing the value of that gift by growing in humility, wisdom, self-control, courage, and integrity.

Purity of heart is about a change of heart from "getting some love" to "giving all love." Purity of heart is growing in unconditional love so you can grow in the other three loves. Some think that purity of heart means "no sex." That's abstinence, a negative impression about sex that focuses on what you can't do and can't have. Purity of heart is the opposite. It's focusing on what you can have, right now: a fully alive life filled with authentic unconditional love and sustaining true joy without regret.

Waiting until marriage to have sex means you are able to grow in the virtues that make marriage last with a pure heart. No, purity of heart

doesn't mean you're a prude. It means you have the
lust by making the foundation of your relationshi
first so that you're free to fall in love for the right, la
no, it doesn't mean you have a negative or unhealth
it shows that you know how much it's worth. You
away for free or for a cheaper value, you're sayin.... .. ..
anything. When you're pure of heart, you're able to focus on being
united for life, not for a few nights.

While many people think having a pure heart suppresses desires, it
doesn't—it expresses your desires in a selfless attitude of true, authentic
love, not a selfish attitude of using each other as objects who can't
express love. What if you're both not using
each other as objects because you're both in
love? Remember Chapter 1? There were many
people in relationships who said the same
thing, but because they had sex early, it
blinded and magnified the problem in their
relationships. Mutual sacrifice builds love; refusing to sacrifice builds
lust.

> **Mutual sacrifice builds love; refusing to sacrifice builds lust.**

When pleasure is valued more than love, you will lose the
opportunity to grow in these virtues. Waiting until marriage to have
sex has allowed me to master myself by growing in these virtues and
growing in unconditional love. At first, the wait was uncomfortable,
even lonely. But as I progressed, my comfort grew and so did my
knowledge of myself, my joy, my self-worth, and my ability to love,
because I was mastering myself. Waiting until marriage is making a
conscious choice to pursue delayed gratification in the areas of life
specifically related to relationships.

Men. Women. if you can be disciplined in your sexual life, there's
nothing you can't do. By growing in these virtues, your sexual urges
lose their power over you. You gain power over them. You grow in the
virtue of self-control.

...NCE IS A VIRTUE, BUT I'M NOT PATIENT

...ll right, I get it. You want sex now. You want love now. You want intimacy. What you really want are the five deepest desires of your heart. We live in a culture addicted to the quick fleeting hookup, the same-day Amazon delivery of pleasure, the miracle cure, and the overnight success stories. Waiting to have sex is the remedy for that addiction. If you think this is just my experience or that of a few others, think again. I'll be showing you the science behind sex in this book too.

Sex is a powerful desire, which is why it can cloud judgement and cause us to make decisions to diminish and not flourish us. The body has a mind of its own. This is why we have to learn to how to tame its desires with our mind. You can't master the nature of love without mastering yourself by having the power over your desires. Denying instant gratification allows you to master yourself by seeing clearly,

> *Self-control and patience mean you order your sexual desires according to the demands of real love.*

making better decisions, fulfilling the deep needs of your soul, creating a higher self-esteem, and dealing with anger and other negative feelings more productively.

Self-control and patience mean you order your sexual desires according to the demands of real love. Real love is wanting the good for someone no matter the sacrifice. Being willing to make heroic sacrifices to do what's best for them and lead them to become the very best version of themselves, physically, intellectually, mentally, emotionally, and most importantly, spiritually.

When we continuously choose short-term pleasures, we are not only blinding our spiritual vision, but we're also corrupting our willpower,

> *Patience stems from self-control, the ability to endure things and not be saddened by them.*

mind, and ability to make choices that can help us to flourish. Just as fine glass of wine can be consumed in seconds, its richness is only appreciated by the person who savors every drop.

Patience stems from self-control, the

ability to endure things and not be saddened by them. You have to learn how to control your impatient desire for intimacy with patience, otherwise you will be dependent on pleasure in order to feel close and, before you know it, your relationship is only based on sex, which will rob you of the opportunity to be fully committed to each other.

Instead of doing what feels good in the moment, redirect your sexual desires to actually get to know the person you're trying to date.

True love requires sacrifice. Instead of doing what feels good in the moment, redirect your sexual desires to actually get to know the person you're trying to date. Instead of building the physical part of your relationship (eros), which can be done anytime, build the emotional and the spiritual aspects before it's too late and sex clouds your judgement, forcing you to stay in a relationship only based on feelings. When you awaken love before its time, you can cause a lot of damage to your self-worth. Don't sell your pearl until it's the proper time.

So what do we do? Who do we trust? Are we all screwed? Did I just leave you paranoid for the rest of your life? Yes. That was the plan all along. I'm a bitter man so I want you to be bitter too. You fell right into my trap, mwa ha ha. You're screwed. I was the evil guru all along.

Relax. I'm just playing. Duuuhhh. Here's the deal, though: you actually are in trouble if you haven't understood that you can't give what you haven't received yet, nor can you receive if you do not know how to give. You can't think you have unconditional love if you've never actually received it. The four love types are all intertwined. So the question is, how do you receive unconditional love at its fullest capacity? What are your thoughts? We'll be visiting this more in Section II in my book, but for now, let's go over the beautiful lies of love.

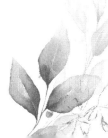

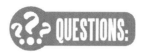 **QUESTIONS:**

1. How do you know what unconditional love is? How do you receive unconditional love at its fullest capacity so that you can give it? (This question is so important, I asked you twice!)
2. What's the foundation of your current or previous relationships? Is it sex? If you're not in a relationship, how can you prepare to live out the four loves?
3. Do you know of any relationships that seem to have all four types of love? What can you learn from them? What can you learn from failed relationships that don't have them?

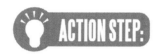 **ACTION STEP:**

1. Read this chapter again and make a list of what agape is. As you continue to read, add to this list. Feel free to message me your thoughts at <u>coachanthonysimon@gmail.com</u>

7

Beautiful Lies

By now you've heard me use the term 'beautiful lie' pretty often, but what exactly is a beautiful lie? Well, just in case you're not believing a beautiful lie about the beauty of beautiful love, I made another beautiful story for you. Beautiful, right? (This actually made me laugh as I was writing it; how beautiful. All right, I'll stop.)

A harmless seed knocked on the door of your house one day and asked you if it could plant itself right in front of your house. The seed said, "Hey, I was wondering if you could dig a small hole and plant me here at the front door? My parents abandoned me and I have no other place to stay. This is the only place I have left. Oh yeah, you don't have to worry about watering me, either. The rain and sunlight will take care of me. So, it's going to cost you nothing and when I grow, I'll give you the juiciest, brightest oranges and lemons. I'll be sure to produce a lot of fruit for you so you can give some to your friends and everyone will love you. You'll be doing all of us a favor."

Moved by compassion, you see no harm in this request and decide to plant the seed. Years pass by and you collect the fruit and everyone around you knows you as 'the fruity neighbor' who dropped their full-time day job to make a living off selling the fruits that the tree promised. One day, you were making your way back home from signing a contract with a dealer and were startled to find your house completely dismantled. In just six hours, the seed had expanded its roots all over your house and broke the water pipes, which caused your house to flood. You're left with nothing but an uninsured broken house, empty promised contracts, and a broken heart full of regret.

A beautiful lie is exactly what it sounds like. It's a comforting lie that seems harmless on the outside, but when examined on the inside with the truth, it's exposed as an ugly life-sucking lie that leads to a dead end full of darkness. It's like the inspector you read about in the previous chapter, but more smooth, welcoming, loving, and deceiving.

Beautiful lies come knocking at your door offering nothing but empty, false promises. Beautiful lies promise you love in a relationship but instead give you lust. You may indeed get pieces and glimpses of love in the beginning, but the moment you get comfortable, you're left with nothing but a broken heart, crushed spirit, feelings of worthlessness, shame and low self-esteem. What was promised only lasted for a quick couple weeks or even months.

All beautiful lies have a piece of truth to them, which is what makes them so believable.

You may be living half of a truth, which is why you refuse to let it go. I don't blame you. It sounds so convincing and it seems like all of the facts are pointing toward it being the truth when in reality it's not. Heck, you may hear a beautiful lie that has 99 percent of the truth and because it sounds so good, you don't realize the 1 percent that's not true. By that time, your emotions have already been stirred up, and you become emotionally invested to give them your trust, worth, and foot in the door. This is why it takes someone who has been deceived himself or who already knows the truth to help you realize it, too. I hope I can be that person for you in this book.

Beautiful lies get you to rely on your emotions and feelings. They're

All beautiful lies have a piece of truth to them, which is what makes them so believable.

smart enough to know that if you don't inform your mind with the truth, your heart will be led astray with the lies they've been feeding in your mind.

WHAT ARE YOU FEEDING YOUR MIND?

What you believe, you live out. If you can believe it, you can be it. Whether you're believing in a lie or a truth, it doesn't matter because the principle stays the same. The brain doesn't know any better; that's why you have to direct it. If you don't enter the coordinates in your mind, they will be entered for you, taking you somewhere you don't want to go.

If you don't enter the coordinates in your mind, they will be entered for you, taking you somewhere you don't want to go.

Your mind is a byproduct of everything you feed it. And if you feed it the wrong things, your mind can easily absorb the beautiful lies we encounter in our environment, our culture, and our society. By then, you've allowed these lies to shape you without even knowing it. Peer pressure gets the best of you and others, so it becomes hard to muster the courage and stand up for what is true and right. Instead of questioning the system, you just go with it.

In the upcoming chapters, I'll be exposing beautiful lies about sex, love, and your worth by helping you enter the right coordinates in your mind, but be forewarned, I'm going to have to wake you up from your deep sleep. You may be sleeping thinking you're awake. You may have thought you programmed the right coordinates only to find out you were brought to the wrong destination after spending years sailing.

Are you wondering how you can find the coordinates? It's all in you, believe me. You've got the map and the key in your right pocket. It's time to take them out to unlock the coordinates to unconditional love.

But wait. There's a problem.

You've had the key and map in your right pocket all along and you never even knew. Before you learn more about the secrets to getting this vision and bringing it into reality, you must first learn how to free your mind—thinking outside the comfortable box the world, culture, and your environment has placed you in. In the next chapter, I will teach you how to think for yourself through a deep conversation between you and your inner self.

Do I have your full focus? Hellooo?

Okay, good. This chapter is is deep and it sets the whole tone for the book, so make sure to read through it it carefully. Did you catch the two intentional errors I made in this paragraph? I'm telling you, wake up! You're dreaming. You've been programmed!

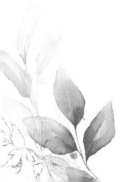

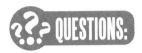

QUESTIONS:

1. Are you open to the fact that you may be living a beautiful lie in your relationship or philosophy?
2. What beautiful lies do you think you're believing in your life?
3. How can you expose more beautiful lies in your life? How can you learn to tell apart feelings and truth?

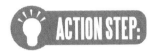

ACTION STEP:

1. Write down what secret frustrations you've had in previous relationships. Write down any time you believed in a beautiful lie in a relationship. Feel free to message me your thoughts at coachanthonysimon@gmail.com

8

Wake Up, You're Dreaming! You've Been Programmed!

Inner Self: Hello? Can you hear me? Hey . . . it's me. Your inner self. You know . . . your consciousness.

You: What's going on? Where am I? Why do I feel so out of place?

Inner Self: Don't worry about that. I'll explain everything later. I don't have much time left before you go back into your fantasy relationship. We have a problem and the king's son needs your help!

You: Uhhhhhh . . . king's son? Problem? You good, bro? This can't be another dream; I actually pinched myself and I'm awake.

Inner Self: It is because you're existing and not living . . . you're dreaming. I'm trying to wake you up. Wake up, you're dreaming! You've been programmed! Look. I've been sent here by the king's son to take a chance on you.

You: What king's son? Why do you keep saying that? Who are you talking about? DUDE! Are you high or trippin' on some sort of new drug? 'Cause even my friends who are on drugs aren't talking like this.

Inner Self: I can't explain now; time is running out.

You: Why do you always have to be so dramatic? I feel like I'm in a movie and you speak such a foreign language, dude. Expresso Englisho?

Inner Self: You are in a movie. The movie of your own life that you're watching right now. We have fast-forwarded your movie to the beginning. The beginning of Chapter 8 of Sex, Love and Worth! The scene where you discover how broken this culture that thirsts for love is and how strongly you have been created to help restore love. Oh yeah, one more thing. I'll take an espresso.

You: Haha, all right, funny guy. I'm not the guy you're looking for. Stop wasting my time.

Inner Self: That can't be true. Before he passed away, the king's son instructed me to write letters to those he will choose. He said that you're one of the people who can help restore and ignite the little love that's left in this culture. He said you have the capacity to find pure love and help others find it too, but he needs you to stop settling and lowering your standards.

You: WHO, ME? WHY ME? YOU'RE INSANE. DO YOU NOT KNOW WHO I AM?

Inner Self: I'm sorry. I know about your past and your desire to find love in a culture that doesn't know what love is anymore. I know you want to find your full worth and be seen for who you actually are. I know this all too well. That's why I need your help. That's why I'm here. I know you have suffered a heartache, growing up in a broken family, and untold amounts of confusion in your previous relationships filled with abuse and trauma. I know you're searching for something that can offer you a greater hope, love, meaning, worth, purpose, and clarity about who you are and what you were created to do in earth.

You: Whaaa . . . what? How did you know this?

Inner Self: Because this culture of death you live in is a ruthless world full of darkness with bullying, gossip, sarcasm, and all the social pressures that make you thirst for praise and affirmation. If you feel ignored or rejected at home, this only encourages you to seek false love and affection in other relationships. You and I are living in the midst of confusion and broken relationships. I'm here to change that. I'm here to restore love. I'm here to allow you to enter into a deeper relationship—a relationship that'll take you to another dimension of your life. Not even another level, but another dimension.

You: Why do you speak like that? Your language is so foreign to me. Dimension? Deeper relationship? Culture of death? King's son? Enough with your stupid philosophical games and just shut up.

Inner Self: I'm sorry, I love you too much to shut up even if you'll mock or get mad at me. You have a problem and I need your help. What you're about to hear will make you mad, but there's no other way to expose the truth and clean your scars.

You: What scars? What is it now? Can I just go back?

Inner Self: Oh, if you want to go back to being programmed you can.

You: Programmed? Now you think I'm a computer. Boop. Boop. Beep. I. Am. A. Machine. I don't know, Mr. 'I Know It All' weirdo head. Culture of death? Scars? Dead end? Dimension? You're trippin'. You've got problems and you need truth, not me.

Inner Self: How can I have problems when I heal them? How can I need truth when I am truth itself? You wanted answers, right? Well, let me explain. The world seems to have lost sight of the priceless worth of true love that flows from pure hearts and innocent souls. Because of this culture of death, people with hungry hearts are exposed, wounded, and starving for the truth about love, their worth, meaning, and the truth about their sexuality. With no pure-hearted leaders to model, no foundation was laid in anyone's lives for how to truly love. Wrong has become the new right and right has become the new wrong. The world is seen as backwards. People are walking with their hands thinking they're walking with their feet. You're seeing with your eyes, but not looking with your eyes. You're hearing with your heart, but not listening with your heart.

You: What do you mean by "I'm seeing with my eyes, but not looking with my eyes? I'm hearing with my heart, but not listening with my heart?" Can I not see right now with my own two eyes that I'm in love? Can I not hear with my own two ears the words "I love you"?

Inner Self: I'm trying to free your mind by getting you to think for yourself instead of the culture of death giving you the illusion that you're thinking for yourself. Think with the facts, not only the feelings. I'm trying to get you to understand that you're looking with the eyes of your heart, but not seeing with the mind of your brain and heart. You're hearing with the ears of your heart, but not listening with the ears of your mind and heart. You can't just rely on your feelings; you must know the truth about your feelings—knowing lust from love, knowing sex at its fullest purpose, and knowing love at its fullest capacity to find your true worth and purpose.

You: But what's so important about the mind?

Inner Self: People like you live in your fantasy world of instant self-gratification for your own selfish, impure desires, oblivious to what is actually truthful by relying on your feelings only and indifferent to truth and finding worth because of confusion. What seems to be happiness is only temporary because evil leaders who brought about the culture of death have selfishly programmed, contaminated, and brainwashed your mind to believe the world you live in is a reality. You may think you're being a manly man or powerful woman when you're actually weak. If they take your mind, they take your worth, value, and identity. They influence you to just follow the system instead of question it. You were created to live fully in love, but instead, you're just existing in partial amounts of love.

You: This is just all too deep for me now. I don't think I'm worth as much as you say I am.

Inner Self: How much longer are you going to be lying to yourself? Since birth, you were designed to be someone with dignity, value, and a unique personality that nobody else has. There's only one of you.

You: But why should I trust you?

Inner Self: Look into your right pocket and you'll realize you've had the key and map Anthony was talking about in Chapter 4.

You: What the heck? Okay, now this is getting weird. How did you do that? I just checked my pockets, like, a couple minutes ago and there was nothing there. How did you put them there? Who are you?

Inner Self: I'm asking you to wake up. Wake up. Wake up. WAKE UP, YOU'RE DREAMING! YOU'VE BEEN PROGRAMMED! Here's the deal. I'm not asking you to trust yourself. I'm asking you to trust me. You're the only one who can unlock that treasure chest that holds the greatest pearl worth millions, but you need my guidance. I can't do it for you . . . only you can do it for yourself. You have free will. You don't have to trust me . . . you'll just be living the same depressing, meaningless, shameful and boring life. Again, you have nothing to lose and everything to gain. Do you want the fullness of love? Do you want intimacy and connection? Are you tired of being lonely your whole life? I can change all that. I promise all those desires and more if you can please give me a chance. Well, the decision is yours if you want to cooperate with me or not.

You: All right, fine. Sorry. What's next?

Inner Self: First, know that the culture of death is run by evil leaders with impure hearts who allow you to have whatever you want by tailoring it towards your feelings and giving you all the fleeting pleasures you desire. They rob you of your ability to think and rationalize and actually become the person you were designed to be—a person worth more than you can imagine.

You: Why wouldn't anyone want me to become the best version of myself? Aren't we all in this together?

Inner Self: They don't want you to find that person because they are bitter themselves—living in denial in their own fantasy world. If you find them, it exposes their fantasy world to others. Then, they lose their business, power, and worldly status, and the truth they've been suppressing comes out and reminds them of their bitter past.

You: Why hasn't anyone ever told me about this? Why have I never realized this before?

Inner Self: Nobody has ever informed or inspired you because they too are zombies walking to their graves of death thinking it's life. This is why I'm your inner self. I let you know you deserve better. I'm the only person left in this world who can love you the way you deserve to be loved. I know that you're searching for the beauty in love. If you give in to weakness by following these cultural models of behavior, in the depths of your heart you'll still desire a beautiful and pure love, leaving you more restless than before. You are capable of heroic sacrifice. Go against the current and shine your light on the dark culture of death, turning it to a culture of life.

You: Why did they choose to do that? Why are they so heartless?

Inner Self: They want your money. They don't want you to live a life of true authentic love and freedom. They have used sex to program these beautiful lies into your heart and mind as 'truth.' They don't want you to experience liberating joy because they don't have access to it. They are products of broken families, broken marriages, broken relationships, and abuse. I tried to help them but they refused to change because of their selfish, stubborn wills, plans, and desires. They couldn't deal with the truth because it was too hard for them to change, so they denied it and made the conscious decision to screw you over. That's their whole life—stealing, killing, and destroying your ability to love and be loved at your fullest capacity so they can feel better about themselves. By never allowing you to fully understand your potential, know your worth, and bring your vision into a reality, they feel better about their own minimized worth.

You: Oooooooh boy. What do I do now? I have so many questions

Inner Self: Oooooooh boy indeed. I'm trying to turn you from a boy to a man. From a girl to a woman. As you keep reading Anthony's book, you'll find the answers to these questions. He is offering you nothing but the truth to free you from the comfortable, beautiful lies you've been programmed to believe in. Before we answer those questions, though, Anthony will be showing you just how precious you are by exposing your wounds and turning your scars into sacred scars. If you don't search for love by finding your worth and raising your standards instead of lowering them, you'll never understand how to love or be fully loved. I'll be waiting here in your mind and heart. Come back when you're ready and you understand exactly how much you're worth and what beautiful lies are.

You: What type of beautiful lies? I still don't fully understand what you mean by that term.

Inner Self: Again, I can answer that question by asking you a question. How do you determine if your current or future relationships are based on love, lust, or a watered-down version of love? Will it last? Do both of you have pure motives or are you merely being used? What is the foundation of your relationship built on? Is it based only on feelings even though you think otherwise? How do you know if you're settling? How much love do you deserve? Can you be having a better romantic life? How do you know there isn't a greater love out there for you? What if you're worth much more than what you told yourself because of what others have caused you to believe? How desirable are you? How much are you worth? How much love do you deserve? How much love do you want? What does it mean to be fully loved and to fully love? How do you find your worth? Just how precious are you?

You: All right, man, this is starting to freak me out. It seems all too true. What do I do now? What's the next step?

Inner Self: It's time to renew your mind. It's time to renew your heart. It's time to free your mind by exposing these beautiful lies about what you believe love is and isn't. My job is done for now. I'm going to pass you to this friend I know. His name is Anthony Simon and he's a professional speaker on these topics. He isn't the best source of love but he's good enough to write a book on it. His book is called Sex, Love and Worth. Funny plot twist is it's in your hands right now. It's like we've met before and I'm more than just a made-up story and character in a non-fiction book about finding love and your worth. I'm actually inside you, waiting for you to read my story, and this isn't a dream. I am your consciousness. I am your mind. I am your heart. I am the pearl. I am your inner self.

You: All right, that's just too deep for me right now. I thought this is a book on love?

Inner Self: It is, and this is the first step. We're using your mind to think. The more you train it, the stronger it becomes. Love starts with the desire to want to love and be loved at its fullest capacity. But we must first inform the mind and heart what love is and isn't. A single idea can change your whole life. Everything starts from the mind. I'm trying to wake you up. Read it it carefully. Anthony will walk you through exposing the beautiful lies and you'll learn more about authentic love. For now, I have to go. The king's son said this is all I'm allowed to share with you right now.

Inner Self: P.S. I wasn't joking when I said, 'Read it carefully.' Go back to the sentence and you'll see the intentional error I made (I added an extra it). Be on your guard with the eyes of your mind and heart wide open, otherwise you might miss something and it could be too late to succeed on the path to finding authentic, everlasting love.

You: King's who? What son are you talking about? What king is this? Man, how much more mysterious can this get? Hellooo?! Helllooooooooooo? Whe— Wher— Where did you go?

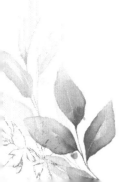

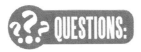

QUESTIONS:

1. What did you learn from the inner self? How do you keep listening to this voice?
2. In what ways are you being robbed of true love? How can you expose lust?
3. Is the new dimension of love worth taking a risk? How can you renew your mind and heart?

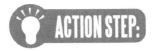

ACTION STEP:

1. Write down ways media creates false portrays of love through movies, books, porn, social media, shows, etc. Feel free to message me your thoughts at coachanthonysimon@gmail.com

9

The Science Behind Sex

I got to confess something: although I majored in biopsychology at the University of California, Davis, science was still boring to me. It only became fun when I started learning about these love chemicals and how they affected my relationships. I'm excited to share with you what I learned. You ready?

Remember the quotes about sex, love, and worth from Chapter 1? Ever wondered why they felt that way and said those negative but true things based on their experiences? There's only one way to find out. Let's get down to the science about sex.

Scientifically, we know that sex engages us hormonally, neurologically, and psychologically; it forms intense bonds mentally, emotionally, physically, spiritually, and intellectually, especially when we do it over and over again.[1]

Again, you know this because you or someone you know has become deeply attached to someone they're intimate with. Scientific research tells us that all sexual activity will affect us on a chemical and emotional level regardless of whether it goes all the way to intercourse or remains as basic as holding hands.[2] Whether it's masturbation and pornography, oral sex, anal sex, vaginal sex, grinding, and even kissing, the brain receives the same information and it interprets the stimulation in the same way it would with sex and releases reward and pleasure hormones and chemicals you will read about later in this chapter that give the "high." For now, this is why you can be just as satisfied having an orgasm by yourself as with a partner. This is also why you can feel so attached to someone you only made out with.

Studies have shown these hormones are values-neutral, meaning these chemicals will bond you the same way whether it's a one-time encounter or a lifelong commitment.

Studies have shown these hormones are values-neutral, meaning these chemicals will bond you the same way whether it's a one-time encounter or a lifelong commitment. It also crystalizes these emotional memories in your mind, making your encounters and experiences difficult to forget, and causing you to fall in love due to hormones.[3]

So, what exactly are hormones? Hormones are chemical messengers of the body that communicate with one another and complete various processes. When it comes to the nature of our bodies, there are three hormones I want to focus on: oxytocin, endorphins and vasopressin.

When these particular hormones are released in your brain, they cause you to bond to the activities, individuals, experiences, or objects that gave you pleasure. Your thoughts are overtaken by your previous encounters, making you never forget who you had sex with or what you bonded with. How is this possible if it was just a casual hookup? How did you fall in love when you least expected it?

OXYTOCIN

The answer is oxytocin.

During sexual arousal, the brain releases a hormone called oxytocin.[4] It eases stress, creating feelings of calm and closeness, which leads to increased trust. Oxytocin works like super human glue because it causes a great emotional bond, increases trust, and makes you less critical of the other person.[5] Research also shows that intense bonding deactivates the circuits in the brain that are supposed to make judgments about another person![6] Oxytocin influences you to focus on the positive while overlooking the risks of relationships. This is why some people will not leave their relationships, no matter how bad the unbiased facts are.

Any of these sounds familiar? "I love them. I know he's flawed and toxic in every aspect, but I love him. You don't understand. Stop judging me and telling me what to do. You don't know me like that. I'm going to stay with him. You don't know what real love is, anyway. I'm special. I'm going to defy the statistics of 80 percent ending in divorce." What about, "I'm not in love, we're just really, really close. Oh, why can't I leave him? Because we're just best friends, okay? No, it's not denial. No, I'm not being used for sex. I go to his house every day because we're friends with benefits." Or perhaps, "Pleeeeaaaaseeeee. DON'T LEAVE ME. YOU HAVE MY HEART! I'll change. I promise. What do you want me to do? I'll do anything!"

We've all heard of people in similar situations to these. Stories like these are more often seen in women than men because estrogen increases the oxytocin response, making females experience more intense bonding than men, and suffer more from broken bonds.[7] For women, estrogen is released during sex and when they give birth to their babies, which is why women love their children and significant others so much.

I mean, I know my mommy loves me to death. She chooses to love me even when she is tired, hurt, or empty herself. She never stops serving me and she is like a walking saint. Just yesterday I was telling her the following: "Hi Mommy, you never fail to love me. You always go the extra mile for me and I see everything you do for me. Thanks for always cooking for me when I forget to cook and knowing what I want before I even know it myself. I sometimes feel like there's a piece of me in you that can connect with my soul." (Funny enough, that same week I found out that research says there is a piece of us in our mothers. LOL! Crazy timing.)

The oxytocin that gets released in a woman's body during breastfeeding or close contact allows her to bond to that child unlike any other love. The chemicals alter her brain to nurture, comfort, and protect the baby. I'm twenty-two and my mother still sees me as that baby. Moreover, studies show that oxytocin can be released by a number of different activities that aren't only sexual but also psychological and emotional.[8] This is why you could bond to porn, a fantasy or imagination, or even just by thinking about someone over and over again.

> **When you have sex, the connection is so transcendent that it joins you and your partner body to body, soul to soul, and spirit to spirit.**

Scientists have explored why these chemicals were created and what their purpose is. It's been said that the "love hormone" (oxytocin) is released to help married couples persevere with fidelity during tough times. These hormones would cause married couples to feel devoted, loyal, possessive, and willing to suffer anything for each other. Marriage is known to get hard at times, so these hormones were instilled in our nature to override feelings of giving up or quitting.

You can't take an orgasm and leave the bonding. You can't take an exciting encounter and leave the memories behind. You can't take a one-night stand and leave your heart, soul, mind, and spirit behind. When you have sex, the connection is so transcendent that it joins you and your partner body to body, soul to soul, and spirit to spirit. Sex alters your brain chemistry and changes you forever by forming an unbreakable attachment with another. This is what's known as a soul tie.

> **Whether you're married or not, when you have sex, your body is saying, "I give ALL of myself to you, babe, and only to you forever, nobody else.**

As a double major in biopsychology and communications, I learned one of the most game-changing facts. You ready? Just as people speak a language with their words, they also speak a language with their body.

Whether you're married or not, when you have sex, your body is saying, "I give ALL of myself to you, babe, and only to you forever, nobody else. Here's everything I got. Here's my pearl. Yup, this is for you and you alone. Let's make a covenant that we will be the only ones we have sex with for life. There's nothing of me that I'm not giving you. I'm giving you my whole body, mind, soul, spirit, past, present, and future self. Let me release these chemicals so we can make that covenant and seal together for eternity."

You see, your body was created to operate under strict neutral rules. It doesn't know if you're married or not; it will still speak the language of love it was designed to speak. And the body doesn't care whether your mind is speaking the same language or not. It will release the same endorphins and chemicals, and continue to speak, saying, "I give myself fully to you."

When you break up, your body is saying, according to nature, "Stay. Don't leave. We're meant to be together forever." No matter how hard you try to suppress these feelings, you can't. They'll come out harder or eventually you'll become desensitized to them.

Do you now see why relationships that don't last can feel like a literal part of your heart has been ripped away? Emotional heartbreaks are one of the deepest pains one can experience. Take it from me. I didn't want to live when I got cheated on. I wanted it all to end. This is why people cut themselves or even commit suicide. The pain of being heartbroken is much greater than the pain of being physically hurt or even dead. When you give so much of your pearl to another individual, you are left with no more value, and no understanding of love or even sex.

ENDORPHINS

Our next hormone is endorphins: dopamine and serotonin. These chemicals are your "happy, rewarding" chemicals that cause an intense rush of pleasure and increase your ability to focus and concentrate. When you do something that excites you, dopamine is released, giving you a rewarding, exciting, thrilling feeling. The more you feel this exciting feeling, the more you seek it. Dopamine is necessary for basic functioning because it gives you the necessary boldness to take risks. It helps motivates you to do everyday things like brush your teeth, shower, or eat.[9]

Dopamine and serotonin are important because when you have sexual encounters or make bonds with your imagination, the chemical release in your brain allows you to feel rewarded, and makes you want to do it over and over again.

When you experience an orgasm, your brain floods with hormones that tell you to do whatever you did again. You condition yourself to build a dependency on that activity for pleasure as you repeatedly do it and do it and do it and do it one more time . . . oh yeah, one more time. Now you see why people struggle with addictions, waiting until marriage, or moving on from previous relationships? It's natural to desire pleasure, but we should control pleasure—it shouldn't control us.

Again, since the chemicals released are values-neutral, the brain cannot differentiate between sexual activities that are meaningful and those that are insignificant. That's why, when it comes time to build a bond, you have no glue left to stick with someone else.

So why was this reward chemical made? Imagine going to the bedroom feeling rewarded and wanting to repeatedly return to that person. This kind of intimacy was intended to be shared with one person only so the chemical reaction could have the strongest effect, not to be turned into a watered-down version. When you're married and having sex with your spouse, you would crave the pleasure of connecting deeply with your spouse not just on your honeymoon, but your whole life.

VASOPRESSIN

Dudes. Ever wonder why you get jealous? Women, ever wonder why your men are so protective? Our last hormone is vasopressin. Vasopressin creates a desire to be committed, loyal, and responsible in a relationship. This last hormone is very similar to oxytocin, except that it is primarily released in the brain of men.

When vasopressin is released and relationships don't last, things get bad . . . really bad. You've seen this when a man falls for a girl and she leaves his life. Some girl becomes a guy's world and he feels entitled to her, as if she belongs to him. If she goes with another guy, he gets all hypersensitive by using manipulative tactics, absurd threats, or unethical ways to control her or the guy.

Why was this hormone created? Survival of the fittest. In marriage, a man needs to have a bond to a woman during intimate contact to protect her and the children from any harm.

PUTTING IT ALL TOGETHER

Sex is not just a mere physical act; sex is a total giving of your best self, physically, intellectually, mentally, emotionally, and spiritually.

After doing tons of research through videos, books, the internet, reliable accredited sources, and interviews about sex and its power, here's what I found: Sex is the surest way to form the closest bond with someone if done the right way, at the right time, with the right position of heart, mind, spirit, and of course, body. Sex is not just a mere physical act; sex is a total giving of your best self, physically, intellectually, mentally, emotionally, and spiritually.

1. **Physically:** Sex includes some of the greatest pleasures shown through acts and expressions.
2. **Mentally:** Sex is the gateway to activated powerful neurotransmitters and endorphins in our minds.
3. **Emotionally:** Sex is expressed through love, surrender, trust, and sacrificial service (giving of the self) to another.

4. **Spiritually:** Sex is a permanent, bonding act left in our hearts and our spirits. This is called the "soul tie."

Many scientists, philosophers, psychologists, church leaders, and happily married couples confirm that these hormones are gifts meant to create a lifelong bond between a married couple and their family.

> *The more you bond with others, the less you'll be able to bond with that one special person.*

They also say that separating from people is painful because we're designed in our nature to be with one person. The more you bond with others, the less you'll be able to bond with that one special person. You'll keep sticking and tearing, sticking and tearing, sticking and tearing until there's nothing left to stick to. You will become torn in body, soul, and spirit.

The reason you can't stay fully intact when you tear apart is because you've invested your mind, heart, body, time, feelings, experiences, and innermost parts of yourself with another. You've given away pieces of yourself that you can never get back. By exchanging pieces of yourself with another, you'll always have a piece of them in you, attesting to the fact that you weren't meant to leave them. You're playing with nature's chemicals, acting like everything's all good. But is it? Is it just a mask you've been wearing your whole life? Has the mask become your identity because you fear rejection? At the end of the day, when you are in your room all alone when nobody can see you, is it really all good? How about when you look at yourself in the mirror after being used by someone you thought was the one? Is it all good now? Is sex really that casual? Let's find out in the next chapter.

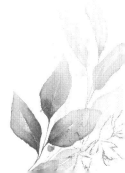

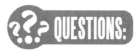

QUESTIONS:

1. What are your thoughts on the three hormones related to the nature of your body? When have you experienced them?
2. Which examples can you relate to? Do you desire to change? What can you do?
3. What are your thoughts on sex now? What were your thoughts on sex before?

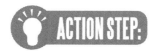

ACTION STEP:

1. Write down experiences when you've seen all 3 hormones work in your life. Feel free to message me your thoughts at coachanthonysimon@gmail.com

10

The Beautiful Lie: Sex Is Casual

Ring . . . ring . . . ring! Are you going to pick it up? Sex is calling and it wants you to listen to this story.

I remember doing laundry a couple weeks ago. I forgot to take some tissues out of my pocket so they stuck onto my black pants. To get the lint off, I used Scotch tape because I didn't have a lint roller. As I taped the tape on the parts of my pants with lint and collected the tissue pieces, I couldn't help but notice that the more times I ripped the tape off, the less value the tape had—it lost its stickiness. Instead of being its original clear color, it collected not only the lint but other pieces of the black pants, making it dirty. Not only were those pieces stuck to the tape impossible to get rid of, but the tape lost its ability to stick to the black pants. I tried sticking it on the wall and it still wasn't able to stick. It lost its value and worth.

When you have sex, you're giving away parts of yourself that you can never take back.

Did you catch what I'm trying to say? Having sex is a lot like sticking the tape to the pants. When you have sex, you're giving away parts of yourself that you can never take back. It also works the other way around: You're receiving parts of another individual that you can't ever get rid of. No matter how hard you try to get rid of the lint, you can't because it is stuck to the tape. Other than the obvious diseases and unwanted pregnancies, you're collecting their whole self—physically, intellectually, mentally, emotionally, and spiritually—onto your piece of tape too. Similarly, if you keep sticking and ripping, you eventually won't be able to stick anymore. This is why some of the people who shared experiences back in Chapter 1 weren't able to connect with anyone anymore. They didn't know the value of sex because of lack of information, which is why they devalued it.

What happens is this: When you have repeated sexual encounters, you lose your stickiness. Scientifically, we know this to be true because as you bond and break, bond and break, bond and break, you lose your ability to properly bond.[1] It's no wonder that, when you're finally ready for that new serious relationship or marriage, you aren't able to fully bond. Something is missing and you don't feel that connected or committed and your feelings diminish, not flourish.

This restlessness causes you to move from one relationship to another. All it takes is for you to see someone else a little more stimulating, more interesting, hotter, and more perfect for you, and you're ready to move on in a heartbeat. You're no longer "madly in love" anymore and you will find yourself feeling less excited and bored, reinforcing the idea that sex is just casual. Eventually, you'll lose faith in failing in love again and nobody seems to "get you" anymore—everyone's boring. Why is this happening?

THE CULTURE OF DIVORCE

We live in a culture that is taught to practice divorce. Feelings. It's all about feelings. Our current generation tells us that if we're not getting what we need when we want it, we don't need to stick around. A lack of understanding is what's robbing us from the sacredness of sex, love, and our authentic worth. And it's no fault of our own.

Sayings like "Connect as long as it feels good" or "Try everything before you seal the deal" or "Test drive the car before you buy it" all reinforce the beautiful lie that sex is casual. I mean, how else will you know what you like or don't like if you don't shop around, right?

Maybe you've wrecked relationships and friendships by sleeping with multiple partners, even after swearing that you wouldn't. Maybe you're tired of the empty feeling you get when you wake up next to someone you slept with because you were lonely or had too much to drink, but you just can't stop.

Perhaps it feels like you're on a dark path of discouraging, drama-filled relationships based on only physical attraction because of sex. Whether it was dating everyone in church or partying hard at college, you will lose your ability to fully connect. You may see this right now, or you may see this when you "get it together" and decide to "settle down" and marry only to find out it was nothing special. Again, your stickiness left you. If you're thinking you're different because you come from a church or religious background, think again. Statistically, the church's divorce rates are the same as everyone else's.[2]

> **You may have connected with so many people that you have become desensitized to the power of sex.**

People wonder what the problem is, but all along, physically, intellectually, mentally, emotionally, and spiritually, they've been making and breaking connections their whole life. You may have connected with so many people that you have become desensitized to the power of sex. This is why it is important to protect your purity—spirit, soul, and body.

You must understand that your ability to be pure and save yourself is not just about giving your V-card to someone. That's not the point. The point is to keep your stickiness brand new so that when the right person comes along, you can connect with them physically, intellectually, mentally, emotionally, and spiritually.

You were made for a single special person—your spouse. Don't lose hope if you think you can't "stick" anymore. You may be surprised to find out these hidden secrets nobody is talking about these days. If you don't feel that you have any stickiness right now, there's still a way to restore your stickiness to keep your stickiness intact. Gotta earn it and keep reading cover to cover.

SEX IS A GIFT

Sex is extremely powerful not only when it's used as it was intended but also when it's not. Sex is a gift. Sex isn't just any gift . . . it's one of the greatest gifts you can give to someone because sex is a gift of the self. But WAIT! There's a problem.

Sex isn't seen as a gift anymore. The world tells us sex is just another fun thing to do on a Friday night that gives some pleasure. The world says you don't need to grow in purity of heart through virtues to have a great relationship. You're right; you don't have to do these things . . . if you want a broken heart and a miserable love life. Last time I checked, two half-people don't make a whole person. Two whole people make a full, healthy relationship. So, learn to be whole by finding your worth through growing in the virtues of humility, wisdom, self-control, courage, and integrity.

You know that the longer you wait anticipating a gift, the more value it has.

When you view sex as a gift, everything changes. You know that the longer you wait anticipating a gift, the more value it has. On the other hand, if you keep giving a gift every single day, several times a day just for casual pleasure, the gift loses its meaning. You must first exercise self-control, disciplining your emotions with patience, and redirecting your desires to understand the value of this gift.

When sex becomes causal, done multiple times a day, any time, any place, and any way, it becomes familiar and people begin to fall under the big trap that leads to sex losing its sacredness, excitement, passion, and mysterious transcendent love. You may find yourself saying, "I know everything about sex. It feels great. What else is there to learn? I've tried all types of sex and I got really good and comfortable with it. I don't have any guilt, shame, or blame; all I got is game. It's all good, dude. It's just sex. I can walk away anytime I want. I can have friends with benefits, one-night stands, and multiple relationships. Isn't it my body, my choice? I can do whatever I want as long as there's consent."

Our generation says, "I made no commitment to you, and you made no commitment to me. What's the big deal?" It says, "You'll be able to walk away from any sexual encounter or romantic relationship without it affecting you at all." This is a beautiful lie because we can't get over the lingering feelings of being bonded. We think that we can just give away our pearl, convincing ourselves we're still rich. The truth is that we were built to bond for a lifetime, not separate after each encounter. We've made something sacred into something casual; something holistic into something basic.

Sex is not casual.

The media brainwashes us into believing that sex is just a physical skin-to-skin encounter. But if sex were casual, why are you hooked in the same lifestyle? Why are you still emotional about it? Why do you feel shame, guilt, doubt, insecurity, regret, or even like you're being used? Why, even though you know you're not being loved, do you stay? I thought you were old enough to make decisions on your own and it was all good . . . right?

BODY, MIND & SOUL

Here's the deal: top scholars, philosophers, and psychologists say that you're made of three parts—body, soul, and spirit. You may have never thought of this but you're more than your physical body. All these three parts have needs to be met and must all be understood, protected, and fulfilled. I'll be talking about all three of these in detail but for now we will be focusing on the soul and the body. The soul contains your mind (intellect), will (desires), and emotions (passions/feelings). Your thoughts come from your mind, your feelings come from your emotions, and your determination and decisions come from your will. Your soul is your personality that holds everything that makes you unique. They all are parts to making the whole. You can't have one without the rest.

Your body wants you to know that it will do its function according to the nature of sex, regardless if it's a one-night stand, your first time having sex with your wife, or with a prostitute. Your brain doesn't care; the same chemicals will be released and you can't stop them no matter how much you suppress, justify, or deny them.

Because our soul (mind, will, and emotions) is affected by our body (thank you very much, hormones), not taking care of our bodies properly can cause mental or emotional problems. You cannot separate your soul from your body or spirit. They are all intertwined and work together. An example of this would be how depression is sometimes brought on by a chemical imbalance in the body. If I have a physical injury, it affects my mind, which affects other parts of myself. The reverse is true too. If I have a mental problem, or unfed soul, these unmet desires or disorders will affect my body. Science attests to this. If you try to have one without the other, you are withholding yourself from the very thing you were designed for. You are withholding yourself from being loved, loving, and being seen fully.

People are always surprised to see they can't get over a "casual" encounter. They'll go back to the same relationship they said they wouldn't. They try to suppress these feelings by having more sex. It's no wonder our society is all messed up, thinking love doesn't exist anymore. We're only reinforcing bonds we know we'll break, teaching us that sex is just casual.

We're only reinforcing bonds we know we'll break, teaching us that sex is just casual.

Now, you must understand that it's one thing to know all this information and say, "Wow, waiting doesn't seem like a bad idea anymore," but it's another to act on it. You'll see how hard it can get in the next chapter.

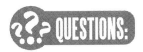

QUESTIONS:

1. What are your thoughts on sex being casual? Where did you first learn these thoughts?
2. How do you think you can restore your stickiness?
3. We're made of body, soul, and spirit. What do you think the spirit side is? How is it related to sex, love, and your worth?

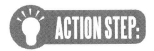

ACTION STEP:

1. Think about some previous relationships you couldn't get out of your mind. Now, write down why. Feel free to message me your thoughts at coachanthonysimon@gmail.com

11

Hahaha, Look! It's the Virgin Boy

I heard it all.

"LIAR! You're not a virgin. You just don't want to sleep with me because I'm not attractive."

"NEEEERRRRRDDDDD! PRUUUDE!"

"Did you forget your chastity belt today?"

"Oh, I get it. You're gay. That's why you won't sleep with me. Well, you could've made this easier and told me."

"If you won't sleep with me, I'll just go to someone who values me enough to have sex."

"STOP! You're being very annoying. Just admit you messed up. We all mess up."

"There's no way you're a virgin. You don't have to hide under shame. The past is the past."

"Stop acting like you're a virgin. You're just looking for glory and attention."

"Oh, you never can get any girls. You have no game. That's why you're a virgin."

"Stop making up stories about having opportunities to get laid."

"Hahahaha! The only kiss you ever got was from your mom."

"You don't love me. If you loved me, you'd sleep with me. That's why I cheated on you."

"You know, girls have physical needs too. You can't blame me for sleeping with another guy. We're not just toys used for emotional support."

"I can't imagine dating someone and not having sex until you're married. You're weird."

"You're not going to sleep with me? Thanks for playing with my heart and leading me on."

"Oh, I'm not good enough for you? That's okay, you're nothing but a tool and a meathead anyway."

"If my body isn't good enough for you, then just say it. You don't have to act like you're a virgin now that we know each other pretty well."

"All right, stop playing around. You can be honest with me . . . how many women have you slept with? It's okay if you've only slept with a couple girls, as long as it's not ten."

"Hey look! It's Mr. Virgin Boy. You're such a man. Yeah right—you can't pull anyone, ya prude."

Waiting to have sex is not pushing down your thoughts to have sex; it's about owning them, disciplining them, and redirecting them to authentic love instead of lust.

I was nineteen years old and all I ever heard were persecutions like these from women and men.

I so clearly remember writing these persecutions down in my notebook (didn't know they'd turn into a book, haha) as my soul was agonizing, crying tears of blood. I felt deeply rejected. I mean, even other student-athletes, teammates, "friends," and women I dated made fun of me for choosing to wait for my future spouse. If it wasn't in front of me, it was behind my back, which was a whole lot worse.

There are many people in this world who will tell you how much you're worth or who you are. They try robbing you of your vision by giving you a programmed version of it, making you think it originated from your own heart.

Despite all this, you must understand that practicing to wait is about the mind as much as it is about the body. Waiting to have sex is not pushing down your thoughts to have sex; it's about owning them, disciplining them, and redirecting them to authentic love instead of lust. It's choosing to discipline the mind and think of the benefit you seek—something that is greater than the desire to give in.

Perfect human love does not require you or me to repress our sexual desires or pretend they don't exist, but to acknowledge the desires and their power and selflessly give it. If we do this, and live out the call to love that is stamped into our bodies, our sexuality will not be something we hide from others, whether we're virgins or not. Rather, we proudly wear it, knowing that special person will see themselves in us.

WHAT DOES IT MEAN TO BE A MAN?

Men and women, I'm talking to the both of you. Whether you're choosing to wait until marriage or not, our society places this standard where we are made fun of for still being chaste and especially for still carrying our V-card. What fills most men and women's insecurities and makes them feel secure is by putting down others and bringing them down. Instead of lifting their significant other up, they bring them down with self-doubt, fear, and blame. I know some people can't take the pressure, so they just want to get rid of their pearls and get the harassment over with.

Some days, I used to lie and tell people that I wasn't a virgin because I was embarrassed and ashamed. If you can relate, why are you ashamed? Why are you letting something special be degraded to something shameful? You wanna be a man? Stop hiding behind your lies because of fear. Grow in courage and stand up for yourself. Be the light in the

Why conform to the statistics when you can create a new statistic?

94

midst of darkness. Why conform to the statistics when you can create a new statistic? If nobody is doing it, why not be the first? Are you going to be a lonely, bitter coward your whole life? When will you ever find true love?

Don't believe the lie that you're less of a man or woman if you don't have sex. Every person who has ever practiced waiting was called crazy, a nerd, a loser. You must break society's status quo.

Being able to have sex isn't what makes a boy into a man or a girl into a woman, because anyone can have sex. It's the ability to have self-control and courage that sets the men apart from the boys and the women apart from the girls. A real man or woman guards their significant other's innocence instead of seeking ways to empty them of it. They lead each other to the arms of unconditional love, not the arms of unconditional lust. Don't settle for less. Stop lowering your standards and allowing fear and your uncontrollable desires get the best of you.

> **A real man or woman guards their significant other's innocence instead of seeking ways to empty them of it.**

A real man is someone who strives to be virtuous. Virtue comes from the Latin root meaning "manly strength." This is why women are naturally attracted to you when you say, "I'm going to work on myself," and you follow through. It's in their nature to go after the most virtuous man.

Check out my vision that got me through these dark moments and feelings of despair in my life.

ANTHONY'S PERSONAL VISION:

Hey babe,

I'm suffering a lot. I don't want to give up my virginity for you. I'm being tempted by all these women and it's not easy. My teammates and guy friends are all making fun of me for choosing to wait for you. I don't care because I care for you more. I'm not going to lie, I feel like giving up right now, which is why I'm writing this letter to you. I want you to know that you're the only reason left why I'm holding on to my virginity. I want to give you my full self.

Let me tell you something: Every day I feel like giving up, I read this letter. I look at it. I cry and clench it with my fist close to my heart to the point I can hear my agonized heartbeat. I want to be committed to you, babe. I want to show you that I waited for you. I don't want to tell you, I want to show you. You and I both know that words are cheap and actions speak louder than words. I want to show you I'm a man not by the amount of women I sleep with, but by the amount of temptation I have overcome by growing in my virtues.

Let my waiting and willingness to carry this heavy cross despite enduring these persecutions show you that I truly love you. I do all this for you, babe. Now, please don't give up on me. I'm sure you're writing the same love letter to me. I'm sure the days you feel like giving up your purity are the days you write to me too. Babe, I got a whole journal waiting for you.

I can't see you now but I hold firm to the vision of what we can be. The vision of us. I dream about it and it sends surging goosebumps from my head to my toes. There's a power inside my heart that says, "You can do this. I believe in you. Don't give up just yet. You're almost done. Come on, it's all worth it. The deep connection you will have with her will be one you've never experienced before. It will be greater than your vision of what it actually is. I know you see it on the T.V. or with that really devout family, but your love will far surpass theirs. All you have to do is finish fighting the good fight, and cross the finish line in the race."

Babe, I don't know when I will see you but I refuse to imagine our relationship suffering because I choose to succumb to the pressure and the temptation. I can't imagine getting into a fight with you and thinking twice about why I married you just because I felt a little bit of pain. No, I'll train my mind for that day by choosing to be pure in heart and wait. I can't imagine our children suffering because they see us constantly fighting. I want them to know that they are loved. I want them to know the power of waiting and fully giving ourselves to them—purity in mind, body, and spirit!

The only way they can know is if we choose to live it. That's what I'm doing right now. I choose to say no to these women in front of me so that I can say yes to you and only you. You see, I'm here on a Friday night and I'm lonely. My "friends" and teammates have just made fun of me for not going to the party with them. They are saying that I'm stupid, making excuses, or an introverted, shy prude with no game. They don't understand what I'm doing but it doesn't matter to me. I know you will understand. I know you're doing the same for me so it's only fair I do it for you. We're a team. Although I can't see those pure sparkling eyes, although I can't touch your soft cheeks and slightly lift your chin and deeply look into your eyes, although I can't hear you say, "I love you, I don't deserve you, you're the best thing that ever happened to me," although I can't speak to you saying, "I'm finally here," I can certainly feel you in my heart saying, "Keep working on yourself. I'm almost there, babe. Keep developing an understanding of what love is."

This is all I need to keep me going. I feel it strongly in my heart. Call it divine intervention from God, or whatever you want. I don't care because I know you're doing the same for me.

Well, I'm getting tired now but I feel better. I offer these sacrifices up to you. Know that I am thinking about you on the daily. I can't wait to see you and surprise you with a love far greater than you have ever received from any human.

Please allow me to be that person to you. Please don't give up on me, because I'm not giving up on you. We're a team and we're doing this together.

I love with you with all my heart, mind, body, and soul.

Your future husband,
Anthony Simon

HOLD FIRM TO YOUR VISION

Remember the end vision: "I like this person and I'm going to do whatever it takes to be with them."

Discouragement comes in when you believe that you can order a life partner from Amazon and have them expedited through Prime shipping in two days.

I know many people's end visions can seem delusional because of the world we live in. Discouragement comes in when you believe that you can order a life partner from Amazon and have them expedited through Prime shipping in two days.

Despite hearing all these persecutions, I held firm to my vision and reminded myself that I couldn't give up. Not yet. She was out there for me and I was reminded of it. I came

98

back to my senses and realized I had to stop entertaining my thoughts to settle. I had to find myself once again.

I always remembered the end vision. My why. My values. Why I believed in what I believed. Most don't know; we're just told. Some of you have sold your pearl because you forget your why or your why wasn't strong enough—it was created by another person instead from your own heart. It's not enough to just say, "I'm saving myself for my future husband or wife." You must go deeper than that, otherwise you will break down and fall under peer pressure and give up.

I thought of my future wife who was going through the same struggles all the time. I wanted to wait for the perfect girl, not the right girl or when it felt right. If you know anything about athletes, they're hormones and blood boil. I burned so badly to want to have sex . . . to want to be so close and intimate with a girl, not just one but many. But through the temptation, I always thought about how my future wife would feel. I always remembered the vision to love and be loved fully. No matter what, it wouldn't leave my head.

It's been shown that surveys of over one hundred thousand people reveal that married couples who go to church—and especially those who enter marriage with little or no sexual history—have the most satisfying sex lives.[1] If you think sleeping around will prepare you to be a better spouse, the evidence says the opposite.[2]

I couldn't have imagined having those awkward conversations with my wife. I couldn't imagine giving her 99.999 percent of myself to her. I wanted to give her 120 percent. I didn't want my hormones to be all jacked up. I wanted to let her know my love for her because I didn't sleep with anyone. I wanted to set a good example for my kids and the generation to come. I couldn't imagine the guilt I'd feel for knowing right from wrong but choosing wrong still. I couldn't live in regret like so many stories and people I heard about. I knew better. They don't know, and yet still have to face consequences. How blessed and fortunate I was to know, so I'd better remain, you know?

I wanted to give my body as a gift to her. I offered it up for her in the weight room, eating healthy foods, respecting my body parts, and more. I always reminded myself, saying to her, "Baby, I don't have to tell you I love you. I'll show you. Words are cheap and actions speak louder than words. I've been waiting my whole life for you and it was hard but I always imagined how great our love would be if we both passed the test."

The more emotional I made the connection, the more real it became.

I stepped into the future and imagined what it would feel like to show her I truly loved her and see that expression on her face. The more emotional I made the connection, the more real it became. I knew life and death are in the power of the tongue so I spoke my dream into existence. Every time I thought about quitting and lowering my standards, I reminded myself of this vision I created.

When I decided to be pure as a young man and to save myself for my future spouse, I knew that I wasn't living for the present, I was living for the future. I made an investment knowing that someone was waiting for me. This is what kept me grounded every day. I knew that to deny myself instant gratification and sex with these surface-level beautiful

Every time I thought about quitting and lowering my standards, I reminded myself of this vision I created.

women, and to enduring persecution, my story was that much more powerful, making me increase the value of my pearl. I woke up to my future spouse every day, believing that she would be right next to me, and now finally I wake up to a real picture of her.

I have found that special person. Will you?

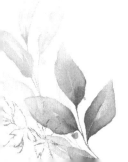

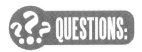

QUESTIONS:

1. How much pain are you willing to take for your future spouse? Seeing my vision, do you now have a new or improved vision?
2. Do you remind yourself of your vision (including all five senses) when you are tempted to give up?
3. What were some examples of people peer-pressuring you to get rid of your vision? Have you let them snatch your pearl?

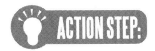

ACTION STEP:

1. Come up with your own vision to review every day you feel discouraged. Be as detailed as possible and put it where you can see it every day. Email it to me at coachanthonysimon@gmail.com

12

The Beautiful Lie:
Everyone Is a Winner—Even Losers

I knew a girl who had a vision of remaining a virgin until marriage. As a kid, she wrote down her vision: "I'm waiting to give my virginity to my husband in marriage because I love him and want to give him my full self." Years later, her mother was putting her socks back in her daughter's drawer and found her old vision. She wept as she knew it was just ink on a piece of paper—it had become a dead vision. Her daughter had given in to peer pressure and slept with multiple guys. I couldn't help but cry when I heard this story because I saw how it affected the mother firsthand. This was her baby, who she loved with all her heart. She just wanted to give her daughter the life that she never had. She wanted to make sure her daughter wouldn't fall into the same trap that she fell into as an adopted teenager with no parents in her life.

Somewhere along the way, the daughter had lost her self-respect and chose to quit playing the game. She crushed her trophy to pieces and said, "It's too heavy to carry. I'll break it and glue it back together later on. My husband won't be able to tell." As she would come back home to her mother's house from yet another failed relationship, she couldn't help but cry. Wanted love turned to unwanted lust because she convinced herself that she was playing the right game called finding love. For too long, she would put the mask on in school, acting like everything was okay, but when she got home there were some days where she couldn't help but agonize over her decisions and try and change, without knowing how to change.

Her sobbing mother expressed to me how she knew her daughter was giving pieces of her body to boys and it only complicated her daughter's life, making her daughter more restless, angry, bitter, and lonely. The daughter didn't know what to do as she never had the best influence without a father in her life. The daughter was conflicted. She wanted change but had no guidance anymore.

Who could blame her? While some would call her the "school slut," I say otherwise. She's not a "slut." She's a wounded woman dealt a bad hand who's looking for love that she never got from her father growing up. She's hurt and seeking for love without knowing how to find it because she didn't have the best upbringing and relationship with her father. Who could blame her for being angry that her father left her as a baby? I know I couldn't. In fact, my heart goes out to her because I want her to know she's made for so much more joy and love. She has so much more worth that she's being robbed of.

If only she knew that she was seeking something greater than sex. If only she knew the truth about finding love through the loveable laws of love. If only she knew she was worth so much more than what the programmed culture of death offers. If only she knew. . . . If only she knew how much her mother loved her. If only she knew.

WOMEN. MEN. IF ONLY YOU KNEW.

How could this story not move you? This story was the final tipping point for me to write this book and publish it after a year of thinking otherwise. We can all relate to this story at some point in our lives. I've shared this story even with the most hardened hearts and it moved them deeply. I can't blame anyone who is a so-called "loser." Who am I to judge their past? Who am I to judge them? I don't know what they are going through. I don't know if they were ever instructed right from wrong. I don't know if they ever had parents who told them, "I love you. You look beautiful. I'm proud of you." I don't know if they were shown physical affection from their parents. I don't know. But I do know one thing: It's never too late to start that vision again. You can have some of the best relationships because you know the consequences of those actions. Believe me, I know some of the best relationships came from some of the most broken pasts. Don't give up. It's not too late.

> **I know some of the best relationships came from some of the most broken pasts. Don't give up. It's not too late.**

When do people give up? They give up when they play the wrong game thinking they're playing the right game. These people may receive fake trophies, fake pearls, and beaten, worn-down medals thinking they're real, but when they see others with real trophies playing the real game, they are quick to persecute, envy, belittle, and hurt because it reminds them of their own failures. This is what happened to me in the previous chapter.

Most of us believe we're holding on to the real trophy when it's just a fake. This is what playing the game of lust thinking it's love is. You see, most of us are comfortable playing this game because we all feel like winners. We'd rather live in a beautiful lie, telling ourselves, "I'm a winner. I'm in the best relationship even though I know I want more." Because these people deny the reality of the situation out of fear or laziness, they end up continuously playing the wrong game, missing the mark, never realizing how to actually play according to the rules of the real game.

Since everyone else talks about this wrong game, everyone begins to play it because it becomes the "swaggy" game to play. You ask around and many say, "I've seen the prize, it's a shining, huge trophy." You may have followed along, not knowing the end prize is actually a rusty, worn-down, cheap trophy of disappointment, heartbreak, low self-esteem, shame and insecurity.

Are you starting to see how popular culture causes innocent people to buy into these beautiful lies and lead others to a dead end as well? For most of us, it's no fault of our own. Just look at the prizes they are getting. But it doesn't take much to find out they truly aren't happy.

WHERE DOES PURE PRESSURE COME FROM?

The problem is there's peer pressure to play the game everyone's playing because if you do, you'll be seen as normal. I've seen many of my friends succumb to peer pressure and their sex drives by sleeping with anyone, which caused them to lose their self-respect, worth, and identity, and wonder why nobody else respects them . . . besides, of course, those living In the same controlling passions of lust and soul-devouring insecurities.

When these friends or people I talk to finally find special relationships, they have nothing special to give their partner because they are all used up. They're only reminded they lost the game, making them a "loser." After they get dumped because they're not meeting the needs of their significant other or themselves, all that's left is guilt and another missing piece of their heart, leaving them hungrier for love and romance them before.

Their passion to find wanted love has turned into pain to find unwanted lust. Exciting nights turn to lonely nights. Candid feelings turn to cursed feelings. They begin to hate relying on feelings because they always are let down by them.

Not knowing how to change or where to even start, they condition themselves to think this is how love is. So they say, "Screw dating. There's no such thing as love; it's all a façade. Everyone's fake so I might as well be fake and use people too because at the end of the day, I'm just going to get used. People with pure hearts don't exist anymore."

Regret eventually gives way to denial and they numb their pain by putting others down to make their beautiful lie believable. They can't see a flourishing relationship or those striving for one because it reminds them of their deepest, darkest wounds. So, they pressure you saying,

> **There are many reasons why we don't act, but the greatest is not wanting to take personal responsibility**

"You won't be a man or a woman if you don't sleep with anyone. Get with your virginity done with already. You'll never get anyone to stay with you if you don't entertain them now."

Everybody wants the good romantic life but not everyone is willing to follow the universal truths all flourishing relationships demand. Sorry, but in order to know and feel love can make you happy, you must follow these rules. It's only a matter of seeking harder. There are many reasons why we don't act, but the greatest is not wanting to take personal responsibility—we want somebody else to do it for us. We're comfortable being comfortable when we should be comfortable being uncomfortable. We're comfortable following the crowd out of fear and laziness.

WHY DO PEOPLE PUT OTHERS DOWN?

You saw the persecution I endured in the previous chapter. Why did it get that ugly? These people can't bear to see others hold on to their trophy when they already crushed theirs to pieces. They view it as a sign saying, "I'm better than you, ya loser. You can never be a winner like me. It's too late. You failed." So they see it as a challenge to try and make the winner a loser too.

What people like this fail to realize is that's not the mentality of the winner holding the trophy. Rather, the winner is trying to help you get back in the game and compete again. Many refuse the winner's offer because it sounds too good to be true. You may hear some people saying or expressing at a subconscious level, "Why would they want me to play when they are the winners? I'm nothing. I'm worthless. I can't be pure again. I already lost my virginity." So, they continue to remain a loser and instead drag others down so they don't have to feel bad about themselves confronting their regretful past. They don't want to be reminded of the bitterness associated with the past so they'll do anything to avoid it. Even remain a loser.

WHY I HOLD ON TO MY VIRGINITY

Remember in Chapter 5 I talked about winning the section championship and receiving the trophy? One beautiful lie the world conditions us to believe in is that everyone is a winner—even losers. What these people also fail to realize is that it's not the trophy that gives the game value, but it is the game that determines the value of the trophy. Some trophies have greater value than others because they have greater stories of sacrifice and heroism. How can a trophy or certificate have any value if it doesn't have a story to it? Thus, the significant value of a trophy isn't the trophy itself, worth $3.33 off an online store, but the story it represents. Without the story, it's a piece of plastic or metal.

These trophies, like our section championship trophy, are only meaningful because they represent a life of virtue, disciplining and controlling our emotions through daily sacrifices: self-denial, delayed gratification, patience, surrender, servanthood, courage to face your fears and doubts, going against the current, and finally, holding firm to the vision daily with integrity, no matter what emotions you experience.

I choose to think with my vision as my priority, not my emotions.

If you didn't understand what I'm implying, the section championship trophy represents overcoming a lot of obstacles, temptations, and insults while choosing to live out my vision waiting to have sex until marriage. I understood that I must discipline my emotions and control them, otherwise they would control me. It's a constant battle but I choose to think with my vision as my priority, not my emotions.

My virginity is a sign of carrying my trophy to my wife. I hold on to my virginity not because I feel forced to but because of the story behind doing so. I know so many people who don't carry their trophy in their hands. Instead, they put it on the shelf where it collects dust, never making a deep emotional connection to the meaning of their stories.

Are you getting this? Anyone can give away something expensive, but only those who understand sacrifice by cultivating their vision and finding their worth can give away something valuable.

It's not possible to make everyone number one, but the world still finds a way by handing trophies with no value to everyone, including losers. Not everyone is going to fall into deep, life-transforming love because not everyone chooses to hold on to their story. You can fool yourself that you still have a story but deep down in your heart, you'll still be restless. The world tries making you feel good, appreciated, and valued by feeding your mind with beautiful lies that say, "You're a winner. You will find pure love too," even when you know in the depths of your heart you're a loser because you don't have a story that supports you being a winner.

THE GAME CALLED SEXUAL PURITY

It's sad to say, but you and I live in a fantasy world where nobody prizes sexual purity. The game of "keeping your virginity" or "saving sex for marriage" isn't being played anymore because it's gone out of style. Anyone who plays that game is "outdated" and seen as unhealthy, weird, or flat-out delusional. Whether they realize it or not, these people are saying, "I'm not worth much." Others believe in the lie that if they lost their virginity, they can't be worth anything. These are lies from the pits of hell. I keep saying it: there's hope. Just promise me you'll keep reading.

There are others that have been born to play the game without knowing why. They were forced to because it was a form of receiving love from their parents or their churches who shoved only negative perceptions of sex in their face instead of talking about the beauty of sex. They've either been scared or shamed into it by an unhealthy fear. Virginity has been shoved down their throats as a religion or cultural practice.

People have stopped playing the game because they don't know there's a trophy with extraordinary value to win. They aren't aware of the rules to the game. Others quit because it requires too much work. They focus on the negative instead of on the positive. They focus on the negative by creating a deep emotional connection to a negative vision, telling themselves, "There's nobody out there for me. I have no value because I'm remaining pure. People define how much I'm worth. It's too much work to be pure of heart, so I might as well give up. Nobody will want me since I'm all used up and dirty. I lost my stickiness. I'm worthless." If these people do have a positive vision, it doesn't last long because they don't understand the depths of why they're doing what they're doing.

> **They focus on the negative instead of on the positive.**

This world you live in has conditioned you to run toward pleasure when you're supposed to run toward what the world calls "pain." Pleasure being a life-sucking, fleeting, manipulative relationship which you put no work into that leaves you more hurt than you were entering it; pain being a committed, intimate relationship you've sacrificed years of your life for, searching, finding, building, and giving pure love.

You see, we want everything right now. There's no more patience and nobody is willing to work for what they truly want in life. There is no perfecting the right virtues of lasting relationships that lead to this freedom you desire. Rather, we're perfecting the vices of decaying relationships thinking we're free when we're really slaves.

Slaves to what?

Slaves to the system called "the culture's world," which you have mistaken to be your world—what you call living YOUR best life—where everything is just about fulfilling all the desires of your heart on your timing and in your ways. This is the world of instant gratification, pleasure, entitlement, and selfishness.

What system?

The system called darkness, which we talked about in the introduction. We're chained by darkness. We're merely living as a shadow under the light of the object presenting the shadow. This is a deeper way of saying that you're not living the best relationship you could be living; rather, you're living a distorted form of an authentic relationship. Or, we can say you're missing the mark. When you miss the mark, you lose sight of clarity, judgement and sound reasoning, making you live in the chains of darkness, pretending it's the light. You lose your mind and your ability to think.

STOP EATING JUNK FOOD

Ever caught yourself binge eating unhealthy foods to cover up your problems? You may pick up these dirty foods and say, "It's just this one time. I'm not addicted," not thinking about the fact that this has actually been their twentieth time. One day, you wake up to take a shower, look at yourself in the mirror, and complain, saying, "How did I get fat? I don't remember the day this happened." Negative self-talk comes in and you try to stop but don't know how. You fail to realize that this lifestyle of pleasure will eventually lead to health problems and even death, with unexpected heart attacks, high cholesterol, and much more. You have to listen to what is and isn't healthy. If you eat too much of one thing, you will get sick and have a headache.

The same goes with pleasure. You can overindulge pleasure all you want. You can avoid growth and contribution, but eventually, you'll have nothing to offer but a heart attack. Stop getting into trashy relationships for the short term pleasure. You'll eat your own worth and story by poising your mind, heart and soul.

BUT ANTHONY, MY PAST HAUNTS ME

Shame is real but forgiveness is ever more real.

So you've got a past? We all do. Get over it. Shame is real but forgiveness is ever more real. At the end of the day, you have the power to feed shame or forgiveness. What will your choice be? Don't allow other people's negative voices or opinions magnify your past. Instead, let the positive voices of unconditional love through mercy and forgiveness magnify your future. Don't let fear kill your vision.

Your past doesn't define your future. If you didn't make great choices in the past, you get to change your future now with your present-day actions. Choice is the foundation of our lives and you have free will. You have the choice to choose to change and become or remain pure in heart, mind, and body today.

You may have had different experiences that have convinced you otherwise: physical or emotional abuse, losing your virginity to someone that never loved you, being dumped, backstabbed and cheated on, hookups full of shame and regret, or even diseases you may still have today. None of that matters when you fully learn from those mistakes. Today is a new day to start your future quest of finding authentic love through purity.

Don't let fear of being rejected—not conforming to the patterns of the culture of death—stop you from actually pursing purity. Fear can hold you back from doing something you know within yourself you're capable of doing. It will paralyze you and lead you to a hypnotic spell of being programmed by the culture.

Can I ask you a question?

What's the benefit? What's the benefit of allowing fear to hold you back? What's the benefit of allowing your past to define and paralyze you? What's the benefit of allowing others to tell you how much you're worth? What's the benefit of giving up on yourself? What's the benefit of not stepping out to life and taking life on? What's the benefit to you? What's the plus in that?

It's possible for you to live your dream, but it's necessary that you associate with winners who are relentless in encouraging and inspiring you to never give up. When the world is saying it's impossible, that you can't do it, you've got to say, "I'm the one. I'm the one who will go against the current and defy the odds." You've got to make it your personal business to make it happen, and you've got to resolve within yourself that you can do it. You can find love and win the game, but unfortunately, even people that understand this formula can't discipline themselves to do it for even thirty-three days. Will you be one of the many who give up during those thirty-three-days or will you defy the odds?

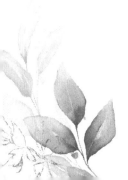

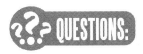

1. In what ways were you like the girl who gave up on her vision? Why do you think she did?
2. Do you have a story of sacrifice and heroism to tell for your future spouse?
3. If not, what fears or beautiful lies are you allowing to control your love life and prevent you from making a change today?

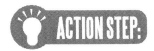

ACTION STEP:

1. Write down all of the sacrifices you've made and temptations you've overcome for your future spouse. This is your reminder. When you feel like giving up, remind yourself of your why. Feel free to share with me at coachanthonysimon@gmail.com

13

The Beautiful Lie: Relationships Complete You

Relationships don't make you happy.

The world is wrong. There is no person who completes you or can make you happy. Sure, relationships might help complement you, but they will never complete you because on a soul level, you are already complete and it's your duty to trace the story of who you are and how much you're worth.

I knew a broken college girl and broken college dude who both had dark pasts and didn't fully confront or heal from their pasts before getting into a relationship. They hoped that this relationship would make each other's souls complete but were disappointed to find out, after a year, that they were more broken than when they started and sex complicated everything for them. You see, no matter what the world tells you, two half-people don't ever make a whole person. You're looking for someone to complement you, not complete you. Two whole people make a full, healthy relationship.

One of the biggest mistakes I made in relationships was seeking my happiness in another person. Another mistake I made was trying to change my partner's behaviors for them. I failed to realize that they had to it on their own; I couldn't be their messiah. Everyone is a work in progress, but so many people don't like to hear that.

Most people can't accept the fact that they can be complete without someone in their lives. This beautiful lie is what constantly propels them to make the same mistake of lowering their standards, over and over again.

> **Most people can't accept the fact that they can be complete without someone in their lives.**

Until you know and love yourself, it's almost impossible to find anyone else who loves you the way you deserve. Imagine if someone came into your life at a time when you weren't ready or couldn't appreciate them because you didn't take the time to date yourself.

IS IT REAL LOVE?

I knew a girl who was waiting to get into a relationship with me. She threw all the signs known to man, but I couldn't appreciate her or even receive her love because I still didn't understand what love was; I was a product of the programmed culture. Because I didn't know myself, I never got together with the one who was meant for me at the time because I wasn't ready to give them a chance.

On the other hand, I was stubbornly convincing myself that the woman I was currently dating loved me. Because I blindly lived in arrogance, I missed an opportunity with an amazing woman. Let me just say this. . . .

Is it real love if you keep loving them, trying harder and giving more pieces of yourself even when you're empty, just magically hoping that they will change or stay with you? Is it real love if you have to convince yourself that they love you or complete you when you still are feeling empty, restless, angry, conflicted, lost, bitter, fearful, anxious, or resentful? Is it real love if they aren't reciprocating the same love you're putting in? Is it real love if it's only based on feelings?

Be real with yourself. Don't live in denial. For many years of my life, I lived in denial, which led me to miss out on so many other beautiful women I could've gotten into a relationship with.

You may have invested so much in a relationship that the last thing you want to do is throw it all away. You may be emotionally or physically married and don't want to divorce this toxic relationship so you keep telling yourself lies: "They're not ready for the label of a relationship. They're afraid of commitment. They don't know what they want yet. They're just going through a lot and they just need more time to figure it all out and I'll help them heal. I'll be waiting right here when they are ready."

I knew several women who told me, "I can't leave him because if I do, I'll be all alone. I fear being alone. I want to be loved and complete." Others have said, "You don't understand—it's only a matter of time before he changes. There's nobody like him. He's so unique."

I've had men tell me, "I've given them everything and I still feel incomplete. How come I'm still lost? Why do my problems only magnify?" Others have said, "I thought she would complete me but I'm only more lost and dug myself in a deeper hole."

You may be distracting yourself with these coping mechanisms and excuses because you fear being alone. You think this is the only way to fulfill your desire to be loved when in reality it's not. You failed to realize that they won't commit to you in the first place because you don't respect yourself. You don't know your worth. You didn't take the time to learn what love is by first loving yourself.

THIS. IS. YOUR. TIME.

Where are you investing your heart and energy in life? You will not have to chase or repair your future spouse. You will not have to compromise or downplay your morals and values. You will not have to constantly try to keep them interested sexually so they don't move on to the next person. You don't have to play mind games or read on all the strategies to get them to finally commit to you and stay committed to you. You don't have to bring sex into the relationship or keep sex as a part of the relationship to have them commit to you. You won't have to convince them of your dignity or worth. The right person will see your worth greater than you see it. They will know you're the catch and will do everything in their power to pursue you—the billion dollar pearl.

You've got to make a conscious effort to begin to work on you. Stop allowing others to work negatively on you. They don't know you like you know yourself. Work toward progress, not some illusion of perfection. How much time do you spend working on you now? In the last thirty-three days, how much more have you learned about yourself? What kind of investment have you made in you?

This is your time to discover who you are. This is your time to discover where you're going in your life. This is your time to take yourself out on a date and find the most stable foundation of self-worth, identity, security, love, and purpose. Don't begin looking for a sense of security, love, or even understanding of your worth in another person. The opinions of others do not reflect your worth.

Stop worrying about being with someone at this stage of your life. You're not going to find your self-worth and identity in that relationship. You've got to stop seeing yourself as incomplete because you don't have a boyfriend or girlfriend. If you don't break out of this mentality, it will be difficult to experience truly healthy and self-giving relationships full of love. Instead, you will seek out the relationship out of anxiety, depression, a need for validation or affirmation, a poor sense of worth, fear of loneliness, fear of rejection, or even for status. You're never going to fill that void in your heart with that perspective about relationships because you'll be willing to compromise your deepest values, virtues, and beliefs in order to be with someone. You've got to stop allowing your self-worth to be determined by how many people you sleep with or what someone thinks of you. Set the bar higher.

I'm going to say it again. . . .
THIS. IS. YOUR. TIME.

117

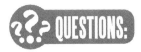

QUESTIONS:

1. Are you scared to leave a relationship because you think you'll be incomplete, unloved, or inadequate? How long have you been telling yourself they will change? Have they changed? How much more pain will you allow yourself to handle?
2. What fears are you allowing to force you into a toxic relationship and deny its toxicity? Have you ever taken the time to reflect and get to know you? Why are you scared to be alone?
3. Do you trust there is someone else out there for you? Why not? How can you gain that trust?

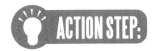

ACTION STEP:

1. Rewrite your morals, standards and virtues. Come up with a plan how you're going to discover more of who you are and what you're in this life to do. Email me your reflections at coachanthonysimon@gmail.com

14

Date Yourself Before You Lose Yourself

I have a friend who has called me several different times saying, "Anthony, I keep getting into relationship after relationship, having sex. thinking I'll find love, and I'm only screwing myself even more. Either these women aren't working out or I'm not, bro. What's the problem? I keep thinking I'll find love and happiness but I'm only more broken. I wish I didn't do this to myself. I need change, man, but I feel like I'm too deep in this dark hole that I dug myself into. What do I do?"

I always respond with the same question. "What are you looking for in life? You want a relationship, so get to know yourself and stop avoiding a relationship with yourself. You have had a dark past and you can't avoid it. Everyone has a dark past. At some point, you're going to have to confront it no matter how painful it is. The more you give yourself to these women, the more you're devaluing yourself. The more you devalue yourself, the more women devalue you and trash you. You and I both know you're worth more than this, bro. You want change? Well, look at yourself in the mirror and start reading the book from within."

START READING THE BOOK FROM WITHIN.

We read a bunch of books nowadays because we want to find out who we are as humans. But we spend so much time reading someone else's story that we don't go inside ourselves. I believe we need to literally turn ourselves inside out and read our own book. You are writing the book of your life every day, but you never read that book because you're too busy reading someone else's.

> *You've been programmed to think there is something defective about you if you're not in a relationship.*

You've been programmed to think there is something defective about you if you're not in a relationship. So many teenagers I've talked with are under so much pressure to constantly have a boyfriend or girlfriend that they never have the time or space to discover their own identity, worth, and innermost dreams.

When you don't find someone on your self-imposed deadline because you're committed to finding yourself instead, it's easy to discard your vision, give in to lowering your standards, and throw away your patience by engaging in reckless behavior in order to force love in your life at any cost. You feel as if everyone else is in love and finding their happiness when it's all a façade.

Beautiful lies start knocking on your door saying, "You're not going to find love if you keep acting like this. You need to change something. You can't keep doing the same thing expecting the same results. Time is running out. You're outdated. Nobody will want you. You don't fit in." So, what do you do? You may compromise and give pieces of yourself to selfish jerks, convincing yourself it's love when you know it's a lie. You end up going for the quick fix of dating someone you barely know, jumping into a stranger's bed, engage in irreversible decisions, and giving more pieces of yourself to someone that doesn't mean it when they say "I love you and you're special."

When will you learn that once you invest in yourself, find the non-negotiable needs of your soul, find your authentic worth, and hold firm to the vision by growing in purity of heart through the virtues of humility, wisdom, courage, self-control, integrity, and patience, things will change? Continue creating a stronger story by creating a stronger vision and living it out every single second. You'll increase your self-esteem for waiting to have sex and you'll discover the person you were designed to be.

Figure out who you want to be and give yourself a lot of time to heal, and discover who you are and who you want to become. What do you want out of life? My friend in the beginning of the chapter didn't recognize women's value because he didn't recognize his own.

You need to find your list within yourself first before you can demand it from another person. Forgetting who you are allows you to become someone you're not. You can't lose the very qualities that made it possible for you to be the catch instead of being the chaser. The temptation is to be someone you're not by lowering your standards and giving in to counterfeits and illusions of love.

> **The temptation is to be someone you're not by lowering your standards and giving in to counterfeits and illusions of love.**

WHO ARE YOU?

Remember, if you don't know who you are, the world will tell you who you are because you'll look to other people for validation. Eventually, you'll find yourself becoming whatever others need or want you to be to fulfill *their* vision of who you are—a fantasy and distortion of who you are supposed to be.

If you live to fulfill someone else's vision for your life, you place your identity on someone else to draw strength and self-esteem from that person. You begin reading their story and not your own. This is why so many relationships fail: You are drawing strength from an outside source and not from your inner self. Your true self has already been written in your heart, but you must unveil that plan and cooperate with it with your free will. Start making choices not to please people but to live out your vision by the standards, principles, values, and virtues that were placed in your heart.

Set your standards high, because you'll get what you settle for. If you need to lower them to date someone, something is wrong. Write them down, but here's the catch. If you write them down, it's only fair you work for them too. Ask yourself, "By the way I'm living today, do I deserve this person?" Tell yourself, "I deserve more. I won't lower my standards because I know what I'm worth and if you can't see my value, that's not my problem nor do I have to convince you. The right person will see it and respect me for me, not my body."

If you don't find out who you are before trying to get into a relationship, they will become your sole source of happiness, love, worth, and identity. Instead of being independent by first learning how to love yourself, find your worth, and root your identity in your vision, you become dependent on something you can't control. This is why so many people who are deep in a relationship experience such drastic heartbreaks and even contemplate suicide. What I'm saying is you may be giving your pearl to someone before you even know the value of it. You have yet to find worth and discover your highest self by dating yourself.

FIND YOURSELF BEFORE YOU LOSE YOURSELF

You've got to find yourself before you lose yourself, otherwise you begin to create a list of expectations for other people to fulfill so you can feel significant, powerful, worthy, loved, and happy. You can't root your identity according to the outer world— the outside self. Instead, you must root your identity from the inner world—your inner self. When you lack a vision for yourself, you become a slave to your emotions and your emotions are easily controlled by the outside world. This is why you have to discipline and tame your emotions with the truth about yourself and your worth so you can know exactly who you are, otherwise you will be programmed by the world.

It's very simple: either you take responsibility to know yourself by doing your research and growing in these virtues, or you allow your physical and emotional desires and other people to control you. Freedom isn't doing whatever you want; it's the ability to do what's right—growing to become the best version of yourself and returning that worth to others. When you have a vision and manifest that vision into a reality for yourself, you become a free person who finds pieces to their identity and worth.

You are free when you're able to discipline your emotions and create your own standards, values, principles, and virtues instead having the world stir your emotions and program you to adopt theirs instead. You can make decisions with integrity based on the right choices because you have freed your mind to think for yourself.

Some of you invest so much time trying to get people to like you that you don't even know who you are. You spend so much time trying to fit in. You know other people better than you know yourself. You study them. You walk like them. You talk like them. You dress like them. You hang out like them. You want to be just like them. You do everything like them. And you know what? You've invested so much time in them you don't know who you are anymore. I challenge you to take yourself out and invest some time with yourself.

> **You've invested so much time in them you don't know who you are anymore.**

You might look cool. You might have all the swag. You might have all the fleeting attention. You might have all the looks. You may have the status, but you know what your problem is? You've been in one relationship after another, yet you've never been in a good relationship because you don't even know yourself. All your energy has been focused on the other person. You spent so much time taking her out. You spent so much trying to impress him. You spent so much time buying her flowers, calling this guy or that girl that you don't even know who you are. You heard what I said: You've invested so much of your time trying to be liked by other people, to be loved by other people, to be appreciated by other people that you don't even know who you are.

I challenge you to invest time in your own self. I challenge you to get to a place where people are envious of you and call you all sorts of names but it doesn't faze you—it builds you. I challenge you to get to a place where you are so secure in yourself that you can walk this world alone. Why? Because you're not concerned with trying to make them happy. All you're concerned with is getting to the next dimension of love. You may be saying, "Anthony, I don't like the fact that you're doing xyz." I'll respond, "I don't care. I'm not living my life for anyone but my innermost, truest self."

Can you say the same? Who are you living your life for?

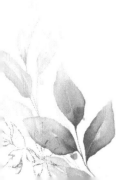

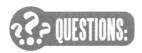 **QUESTIONS:**

1. Why do you continue to read other people's books and not your own? When was the last time you took yourself out?
2. Do you have any wounds you need to heal from or are avoiding? If not, have you suppressed them so deeply that you forgot about them? What have you been distracting yourself with to avoid the non-negotiable needs of your soul?
3. What have you been compromising in your own relationship with yourself? Do you know who you are? Do you know why you're here on planet Earth? Who are you? What were you born to do? Are you scared to date yourself? Why or why not?

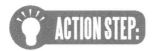 **ACTION STEP:**

1. Go on a dating fast. Spend at least 6-12 months getting to know who you are. Create a plan how you're going to stick to this action step even when you feel lonely. Send it to me at coachanthonysimon@gmail.com

15

The Secret Magic Potion to Finding Love

You: Wait a minute. Wait.

Inner Self: Yes. Exactly!

You: There's no way.

Inner Self: I was telling you. Get ready to wake up. You're starting to see, aren't you? Explain to me what it is that you see.

You: That just can't be. It's deeper than I thought.

Inner Self: Indeed. Now tell me—what is it that has caught your mind?

You: I'm worth more than I thought I was worth. I can't believe I believed the lie that I was just an ordinary human being. How was I so dumb? How did I not know my worth? But exactly how much am I worth? I don't know.

Inner Self: You're starting to learn fast. Explain to me.

You: Without the wisdom you gave me, I would've still been a slave, giving away pieces of myself in body and soul to others to get my worth from them. The key you were talking about that's in my right pocket is the key to unlocking my greatest self and worth that's been hidden in me for so long.

Inner Self: You're learning quicker than I thought.

You: When you said the truth would set me free, you meant it. I feel so much different but I don't understand this supernatural feeling. It's like. . . .

Inner Self: I know, it's like goosebumps surging from your head to your toes.

You: EXACTLY! How did you know?

Inner Self: I wasn't lying when I said I know who you are. Let me explain to you what has happened. Your soul has been locked up in a cage, screaming, "LET ME OUT! LET ME OUT! I NEED HEALING! The more you blocked out that voice by growing your own voice with the fantasy you live in, the more the fantasy's voice overpowered it. Living in your comforting beautiful lies, you've become numb to the truth because you kept missing the mark.

You: What's wrong with my soul though? I don't see anything

Inner Self: Ever went to the doctor?

You: Yea, of course.

Inner Self: Why did you go?

You: Obviously because I was hurting. I was either sick or broke a bone.

Inner Self: How soon did you go when the problem occurred?

You: That's a no brainer. Immediately. The pain and discomfort is unbearable.

Inner Self: Exactly my point. Your soul is sick, dirty and broken. I'm asking you to come to me . . . your doctor. I want to heal you from your wounds and restore your brokenness with my love. You can't see your own soul, but I can since I live in you. Remember, I'm your inner self. So, how much longer will you wait for me to heal your soul and set your free?

You: Whoa, dude, am I trippin' now? This is deep. What did you do to me?

Inner Self: I've been trying to free your mind and soul and I see it's starting to work. This is deeper than you ever could know. The symbolism is deep.

You: It feels so good. This. . . . This is a pleasure I can't explain.

Inner Self: It's called growing in virtue. There are many virtues to cultivate and grow. In this case, this virtue is wisdom—a revelation about yourself which frees you from the beautiful lies. It's the truth that sets your mind and heart free from the culture of death. When you grow in truth, you become a better version of yourself. This pleasure is a pleasure that lasts. It's one of the deep, fulfilling pleasures of the soul. Wisdom. Remember it. Wisdom.

You: Wisdom, huh? Tell me more about wisdom.

Inner Self: Wisdom is like a mother who teaches her children and gives help to those who seek her. Whoever loves wisdom loves their life, and those who seek wisdom are filled with joy because they receive blessings.

If you listen to your mother's instructions, you are secure and will be able to teach others about their worth, love, and much more.

You: Why doesn't everyone inherit wisdom?

Inner Self: Just like a loving mother calls out from downstairs, 'DINNER'S READY!' so does wisdom. She raises her voice, knowing you're far from her. Everyone hears her but not everyone chooses to come down and eat dinner. They refuse to listen to her call because they are slaves to their own diminishing habits, thoughts, and passions. They would rather live in short-term pleasure than lifelong pleasure that takes longer to cultivate.

You: Wow. No wonder Mom didn't give me my grilled chicken sandwich that one day.

Inner Self: Haha. Funny. I need you to focus. Wisdom is also like a mother screaming, "FIRE! MY CHILD, RUN! GET OUT!" She tries to protect her children. Some choose to leave everything and run; others choose to grab everything and run. Those that drop everything and leave don't burn, but those who choose to grab everything may suffer from permanently being burnt or even death.

You: So you're saying that sometimes it could be too late to get wisdom and I may either suffer death or serious permanent consequences because of it?

Inner Self: Yes, that's why you can't live under the mentality of, "I'll worry about it later, because later may be too late." Why take the risk?

You: So why do people not listen?

Inner Self: Just like a beautiful woman with a great personality, face, and body won't just give her virginity to any man because she knows her worth, wisdom doesn't simply give away her precious pearls to just anyone. Rather, just like the gorgeous, dazzling, stunning woman would test a man and see if he is actually worthy of her, so too will wisdom test you.

You: Hmmm. Interesting analogy. Never heard of that before. How does wisdom test?

Inner Self: The virgin girl wants to make sure you're able to exercise self-control, discipline, patience, wisdom, integrity, confidence, courage, humility, and most importantly, purity of heart. To make sure you're worthy of her love, she wants to know without a doubt in her mind and heart that you understand what it takes to conquer your fears and arise as a heroic man who makes sacrifices to provide for not only her but her kids to come too. She does so by setting hidden traps—you hit one and you're out. One of those traps is that she may leave you to see if you're confident that she will come back and that you can live life without her. It's like the survival of the fittest. She doesn't just want any man—she wants the most virtuous man. Very few make the cut, but the ones that do are spoiled and cherished with her exotic, mysterious, flamboyant, compassionate love.

You: Makes sense. That actually happened to me before. Man, those girls are hard to get. I failed her test.

Inner Self: Wisdom tests you by observing how you respond to pieces of the truth. Wisdom will first take your hand and lead you along tortuous paths that rebuke you and expose you to fear, doubt, pain, and discipline. Until she trusts you can handle the pain on your own, she will leave you to finish walking the distance. Some turn back, scared to do it on their own. Others rise up to the challenge, go against the current, and become heroes. Very few succeed. I was told you would, so I'm taking a chance on you.

You: What does it take to be a hero?

Inner Self: Purity of heart. You become pure of heart when you grow in humility. And let me give you another secret. . . .

You: Secret? I can't do this. I'm sca— sca— sca. . . .

Inner Self: "Scared? I know. I know you're scared. To start this process, it takes courage. Courage isn't the absence of fear; it's the ability to acknowledge fear and march boldly forward regardless of what the outcome is.

You: What about humility? How do I get that?

Inner Self: Every virtue flows from humility because humility is the ability to see yourself as you truly are. To know yourself—the very best version of yourself. For now, the four virtues I want you to grow in to find yourself are wisdom, self-control, courage, and integrity. These will lead to becoming humble.

You: I'm full of questions. What is the best version of myself? How do I know how good I am? What's the truth about me? Who am I? What's the book inside me? How do I learn what it means to be loved and love at my fullest capacity? Just how much am I worth?

Inner Self: Wisdom. Wisdom. Wisdom. It all starts from seeking the truth about relationships. What works and what doesn't work. At the end of the day, you have free will and it's all up to you. I can't just tell you the answers right now—it isn't the right time. You must think about them on your own. For what good is it if I just tell you the answers? Every teacher knows that the teacher shows up and teaches when the student is ready to learn. Remember I said wisdom will test you? I am the source of wisdom and this is your first test. If you really want to find the answers to these questions, read part two of Anthony's book. That's the very first step. Keep striving to be the best version of yourself by seeking only the truth about you. For now, I want you to live in authentic love—a selfless life geared toward making others happy. Learn how to be selfless and you will grow in humility. You will know yourself, and when you know yourself, you will find the best relationship your heart has always yearned and thirsted for.

You: But . . . don't you see that I'm serious? I want. . . .

Inner Self: You want to learn. You are learning. Did I not just say I gave you the first step? Trust in me. You're motivated to learn at this instant, but motivation comes and goes. You need to learn how to desire truth at all times, not just when you are happy or sad. Right now you're encouraged but tomorrow you may not be. I might give you too much and you'll get discouraged.

You: That's not fair, though.

Inner Self: You'll thank me later. You're growing in patience and self-control right now. As you're reading these next chapters about love from Anthony's book, keep in mind those same questions you had. We're entering into part two of the book and it's about to get deep.

You: All right, man. I guess . . . I just . . . I just hope this will all be worth it. I hope I can find love.

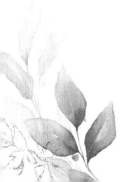

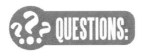 **QUESTIONS:**

1. Do you desire to know the truth about who you are? How can your soul be sick? How can you find healing in it?
2. What do you think love is? Where are you getting this definition from?
3. How are you pursuing wisdom about yourself? When has wisdom tested you in your life? Could it be testing you at this very instant?

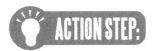 **ACTION STEP:**

1. Write out what stood out to your mind and heart this chapter. Send me your thoughts at coachanthonysimon@gmail.com

PART 2
Finding Love & Worth

16

Strike 1! Strike 2! Strike 3! YOU'RE OUT

LET'S GO, BABY!

FINALLY! I finally found her. Can you believe it? I went around telling all of my friends that I finally was in a committed relationship with the best woman I had ever met in my life. Now, if you know anything about me, you know I don't go out giving that title to just anyone.

Without getting into too much detail, this girl was a beautiful, tan brunette student athlete in college who had one of the greatest personalities I've ever encountered. We just clicked and I felt so loved, understood, and seen by her. I never had laughed and smiled so much in my life. She made me feel like a king and she was my queen. I loved Tiffany (not her real name). I loved her with all my heart. I never felt so cherished by a woman in my life.

> **Feelings come and go but loyalty stays no matter what.**

I remember my cheekbones cramped up because of how much I smiled as I looked into her eyes, feeling so loved and valued. I don't know how else to say this, but all I wanted to do was have sex with this girl. I was very tempted at times but I reminded myself, "Anthony, you need to test Tiffany first. Is this love or lust? You can't rely on how you feel to truly gauge the trustworthiness of a relationship. Feelings come and

137

go but loyalty stays no matter what. You've got to see if she's loyal by testing if this is true love or lust. You can't get the chemicals involved and lose your judgement."

After reminding myself it would all be worth it in the end, a few weeks into exclusively dating her, I made my intentions very clear. "Tiffany, you make me feel so special. You defend me and support my dreams when many don't. You've got such a pure heart and I want to see if our relationship is based on love or lust. I'm waiting to have sex until I get married. I don't know what your past may be but that's where I stand and I hope you have the same vision." She was on board, replying, "Definitely. I have the same values and morals. I really want to get to know you as well and see you for your authentic worth. I don't want to pressure you or myself into having sex and awakening love early."

I was in shock. She was actually on board, as pretty, athletic, fit, funny, popular, and positive as she was. Tiffany loved me for me. She bought me gifts in Christmas season, we Facetimed regularly, supported each other's games, spent time with each other's families, and most of all, kept our relationship pure. All those lonely nights were finally going to pay off. I remember saying, "Tiffany really loves me for me. FINALLY! I found my dream girl. I feel so unworthy with her."

A couple months passed and she drove over to my place early in the morning to go on a hike. We spent the whole day together and I even went bowling with her family that night. She dropped me back to my place at one in the morning in her car and asked if she could come over to my apartment and stay the night because she was tired. I tried reminding her of our promise but something changed in her when she said, "Anthony, I've really been getting to know you well and you make me feel so special. What's so wrong if I stay the night over? Don't you love me too?"

I responded, saying, "Believe me, Tiffany, you're the prettiest girl I know in my life right now. I'd kill to invite you over but you and I are worth more than that. Sex can blind our relationship and cover up some problems you and I may have that we don't know about. It can be a trap."

She didn't understand as she continuously pressured me to have sex with her. It seemed like she had just been trying to win me over by acting like a "good" girl. I think she saw it as a challenge. When I called her out on it, she said, "I just don't want to lose you. I want to show you I love you." I explained to her how I would stay with her if she held true to her promise.

She got mad and left.

Two weeks later, I saw a photo of some shirtless guy at her house posted on her Snapchat story. It was early in the morning and I grew very suspicious. I confronted her about it and she said, "Is what I did not enough for you? You know, girls have physical needs too. You can't blame me for wanting to have sex. We're not just toys used for emotional support."

Strike one!

Strike two!

Strike three!

YOU'RE OUT!

I was cheated on for the third time.

I was nineteen when I pulled out my notebook out to tally up yet another failed relationship. As I looked in my journal, I couldn't help but hide my tears and agony in my pillow. I remember locking myself in the bathroom, screaming, in tears. I recorded myself and rewatched the video recently. Man. It's rough. I was in deep pain. I can't express any of it. I gave my trust to this person after breaking down my wall of fears and doubts only to get let down once again.

I remember screaming, "IS THERE ANYONE OUT THERE FOR ME?"

I mean, how could I have had such bad luck? Like three times! SERIOUSLY?!?!?! I don't know about you, but that's unheard of. Like once is understandable, but three? I'll admit, the first one wasn't the best pick, but over time I had learned the next two were really virtuous, quality women. I was just in shock.

As I cried that day, I remember asking myself, how can I ever find a loyal girl? How do I know if she genuinely loves me for me or not? Is there a way I can test our love? There has to be a way. I had thought this was love. Everything had gone so smoothly. She did everything with me, and I'd even met her family.

It took time to sink in, and my body was in great shock. I was done. I. Was. Done.

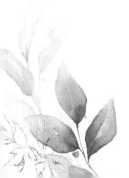

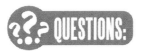

QUESTIONS:

1. What are your thoughts on waiting until marriage even when you feel like she or he is the one?
2. When have you been backstabbed in your life? When did someone's words not support their actions? How can you learn from these mistakes?
3. How did you respond to being played? Bitterly? Did you numb the pain? Or did you forgive?

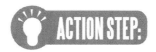

ACTION STEP:

1. Write down why you think I would wait until marriage even when I felt in love. Email me your answer at coachanthonysimon@gmail.com

17

I Lust– I Mean, I Love You, Babe

Wow.

After reflecting on my deep agony, I realized that love can be disguised as lust if self-control, patience, sacrifice, and discipline aren't practiced. Tiffany was saying with her actions, "Gimme, gimme, gimme! Me, me, me! It's all about me. I don't care about your feelings, I'll only do as much as I can to win you over until I find someone better than you."

Sometimes a person's actions may appear romantic because they're so imaginative and thoughtful, but the actions may be done with the aim of manipulating or seducing the other. Again, only when purity is present can one tell the difference between loving romance and selfish seduction. You saw how I told Tiffany that I wouldn't sleep with her and she left me. When that happened, I knew immediately what I was being "loved" for.

Women. Men. If someone has many smooth words to say to you, be careful—it's not always love. Studies have shown that women in particular perceive when they are being viewed merely as an object for another person's gratification. When a woman senses lust in the heart of a man, she feels a restless vulnerability and even resentment. One expert on the female brain noted that a woman's sexual pleasure is greatest only if the amygdala—the fear and anxiety center of the brain—has been deactivated.

It appears to be love because it all feels good, it's spontaneous, and you hear the words from the lips saying, "I love you. Let me just make love to you tonight," but you don't hear the words from the body saying, "Let me use you for my own pleasure. I have needs that need to be met and you're the next person on my list to meet them. Just give me your body so I can drop you like a fly later."

LUST VERSE LOVE

Using another person isn't romantic. It's ruthless.

By practicing to wait to have sex until marriage with the virtues of self-control and patience, you express how sacred sex is and make it worth that much more. You increase the value of your pearl by discovering that rather than inhibiting your freedom, these virtues make you free to love. Choosing to wait brings light into people's intentions and frees you to know if you are being used.

> **Choosing to wait brings light into people's intentions and frees you to know if you are being used.**

You may be saying, "Living without sex until marriage is difficult," but I'm saying, not living with purity of heart is harder. You see the pain it causes in your relationships, don't you? Remember Chapter 1? Love is impossible without purity of heart. Since waiting until marriage protects you from the self-centeredness of lust, it frees you to look beyond yourself and to love in a self-giving way, enabling you to become your fully alive, authentic self.

Lust always leads to self-centeredness. It prevents you from receiving and giving yourself as a gift to others. Lust deforms your vision, making you see others as objects to be used rather than walking, talking, breathing human beings to be loved.

I remember telling a friend, "Once you ignite the flame of sexual desire, it becomes a fire that doesn't stop burning until everything in its path is consumed." Giving in to your uncontrolled hormones isn't romance. It's an addiction. It's lust disguised as the pearl of love, with nothing but hollowness inside. It's the shiny apple on the outside that's rotten on the inside.

Wondering how you can spot the fake pearls from the real ones? Ladies, this next section is for you. Men, you'll also get a lot out of reading it, as this can work the other way around, too.

THE DANGER OF MEN

A famous quote says it best: "Many women give sex to men for the sake of getting 'love,' while the men often seem to give 'love' for the sake of getting sex." Women. . . . Be. Careful. Trust me, I've been to a lot of parties and believe me, seducing women in front of your friends is a game many men play to fill their insecurities or needs by "scoring."

Most men (women too) will make their actions appear so romantic because they are fueled by the desire to sleep with you and increase their body count or list. They'll build you up with the words you want to hear and, based on how you respond, they'll adjust. Once they get you to bite by saying things like, "You're special and have a great personality. I've never seen anyone like you. Your dress compliments your eyes. You're different and I feel a special connection to you," they'll brag to their friends by saying, "Look who I hooked up with." This is why you have to test if he's actually in the relationship for you or not by choosing to wait to have sex. They'll love you as much as you want to be loved. Demand the highest price of love by choosing to wait. Choosing to wait ends all games and protects you from all heartbreaks. You'll save yourself the mind games men play to get you into bed.

> **Choosing to wait ends all games and protects you from all heartbreaks.**

Other men (women too) will get you to doubt your value and worth to get what they desire. For the first example, they'll use fear to manipulate you to do whatever they want. If you don't comply with what they want, they will leave you or threaten to do so. They'll blame you, saying it's your fault, poking at your insecurities and telling you you're not good enough. They claim that they are perfect and you're simply wrong.

Don't believe me? It's okay. You don't have to. Just check out the statistics.

Did you know that 74 percent of girls who lose their virginity as teens lose it to an older guy?[1] That's legit crazy, but sadly true. Older guys have been around and have more experience. They give gifts such as promise rings and say things like, "We will be together forever, so our sex is sacred sex. There's no one like you, babe. You deserve the best." It's all a play on words. Don't bite from the poisonous fruit. Use logic and ask yourself, why isn't he going for women his age? Is he that insecure that he has to go for women younger than him?

Smooth, insecure players use flattery to try and woo you and bring down your intuition, causing you to think, "He's different than all the other men I've met." To most men, it's just a game of wanting to be wanted. Who can get the most attention? Who can get the most "action"? Who can get the most "love"? Don't fall for it when he says, "I've never felt this way before. You make me feel so comfortable. I just want to show you I love you—I'm comfortable if you aren't ready to have sex yet, though." It gives you the illusion that he's willing to wait for you. Anyone who uses their strength to control a woman shows that he is too weak to control himself. He seeks to rule another because doing so is easier than ruling over his own insecurities, pride, selfishness, doubts, fears, anger, lust, and other weaknesses.

Wanna know if someone is bluffing? Wanna know if your relationship is based on love or lust? Wanna know if you're loved for yourself or if it's a trap, like Tiffany turned out to be? Stick around for the next chapter.

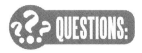 **QUESTIONS:**

1. Have you had any Tiffanys in your life? What can you learn from your mistakes? What can you learn from my mistakes?
2. "Once you ignite the flame of sexual desire, it becomes a fire that doesn't stop burning until everything in its path is consumed." Have you noticed any truth to this saying in your life or in the lives of others? How so?
3. How has lust broken your relationships in the past or in the present?

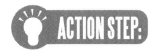 **ACTION STEP:**

1. Write down all the times you've been tricked, manipulated or reduced to a piece of meat. Then, write down how, when and why you let your guard down to these particular people. Was it related to low self-esteem, anger, loneliness, lack of identity, lack of purpose? Feel free to message me at coachanthonysimon@gmail.com

18

The Love Test

Read this conversation about relationships I had with Jeremiah, a friend of mine. (Not his real name.)

Jeremiah: Anthony, I just don't know, man. I keep getting cheated on or dumped out of boredom. How do you find loyal women? I have trust issues with my current relationships I'm in now.

Me: Easy, bro. Have you heard of the love test?

Jeremiah: Love test?

Me: Yeah, dawg. The love test is the surest way to see if the person is actually in love with you or just using you for pleasure.

Jeremiah: Man, you pullin' this out of your butt or something, bro?

Me: Nah, man. This is a real thing. Tired of relationships continuously failing? Got trust issues? Apply the love test.

Jeremiah: Da hell? What's that, Ant?

Me: You wanna know if someone likes you for you or your body? Remove the sex. Looking for a lasting relationship, knowing that you're loved is much more exciting than wondering if you're being used.

Jeremiah: NO SEX?!?!? YOU CRAY-CRAY, BOI!

Me: Anyone who says no to waiting isn't making a statement about you. It's about them. They're trying to fulfill their needs and desires.

Maybe you're like Jeremiah and you're saying, "No sex?!?! You're crazy, Anthony. That's not natural."

NO SEX?!?! YOU CRAY-CRAY BOI

Sex is a gift to another person and we are created to become gifts to one another. You can't find yourself until you can learn to express the power of love by becoming a gift for another person. Human beings cannot be complete without fulfilling the deep meaning of our existence, which is to become a gift to another. One of our deepest, most natural desires as human beings is to fulfill the power of love by becoming a gift for someone. If you understand the magnitude of the gift of love, you understand how sacred sex can be. Affirmation of the person makes authentic communion possible. How could there be a true union between two people if they are unaware of the magnitude of the gift of the other?

> *If a person does not have self-control, it becomes impossible to make a gift of one's self*

A person cannot give what he or she does not have. If a person does not have self-control, it becomes impossible to make a gift of one's self. Instead of making a gift of one's self, the person uses another as an outlet for their perceived sexual "needs." Through self-mastery a person becomes free to love.

Good things are worth waiting for. What was once seen as just passive waiting becomes a period of realization that teaches you how to love. Initially it's hard to stop sex. You're not granting your body the fulfillment of its natural desires, but it's a whole lot harder breaking free from being a slave to sex. Ask yourself these questions: What am I compromising to have sex and what is sex costing me? What am I not experiencing in my life that I might find if I stop obeying my sex drive? Can I make doing what's right more important than doing what feels good?

THE BODY SPEAKS JUST AS MUCH AS THE LIPS DO

Let's use Tiffany as an example. Tiffany got mad at me when I suggested waiting. With her actions, she was saying, "If he doesn't give me sex, I'll stop talking to him and I'll get it from somewhere else to fulfill my desires." Some of you may be in a relationship where that person's body is speaking just as much as their mind is.

Tiffany leaving over sex was a blessing to me because it told me that she wasn't the one. Had I ditched waiting until marriage out of desperation, I would've lost myself. Then, self-hatred would come and I'd become bitter and would've never found the lover I have right now.

Ladies, don't believe the lie that there are only a few good men out there. Believe me, I've seen a lot and know a lot too. Men, don't believe that the lie that there are only a few good women out there. Let them come to you naturally.

If I lived under the lie that there are no women out there for me, I would've lowered my standards with Tiffany. I would've told myself, "I'll do anything to please her so she stays." This pressure would've compromised my morality, my values, my non-negotiable standards, and the vision I shared with you in Chapter 11. It wouldn't have been love. Eventually, I would've resented her for making me be someone I wasn't.

> **Purity of heart isn't the loss of freedom, it's the fulfillment of it. A person who is controlled by their hormones isn't free.**

Tiffany claimed she wanted to be free with me and grow in love, but freedom isn't doing whatever you want. Freedom is the ability to do what's right. We become free and able to authentically love when we have self-control. Purity of heart isn't the loss of freedom, it's the fulfillment of it. A person who is controlled by their hormones isn't free. This is why so many relationships fail and marriages end in divorce because someone wasn't loyal. Lust blinds us and distorts our desires while purity liberates us.

You want freedom? Learn to become pure in heart by testing your love and waiting until marriage to have sex. You won't have to worry about questions like, "Am I being used? Are they being loyal to me? Do they really love me for me or my body?"

So, if you don't want to be cheated on, if you want to find a loyal relationship where you're valued for your true authentic self, not a mask you put on, then you're going to have to practice this virtue that was a game-changer for me.

When I started putting this virtue into practice, I went from dating women who I had to be someone else for and who would end up cheating on me to dating women who would help me become a better version of myself and genuinely love me for me.

The love test is exactly what it sounds like. It answers the question, "Is your relationship actually based on love?" So many are quick to answer "yes" only to find out it was a "no" in a matter of weeks. You saw it in my own life, played out in my experiences with Tiffany in the previous chapter.

If you remove the sex or make it clear that you are waiting until marriage to have sex, you'll know what the other person was chasing you for. You can't be afraid that someone will leave you unless you give them something sexual. Let that person be afraid that they will lose you unless they learn to see your worth. You're not just another date, you're a soulmate. Don't compromise your standards for a little fleeting attention by giving in to what someone wants and ending up feeling used, lonely, and emptier than before. You can't live in fear of staying alone for the rest of your life. When you value yourself and put a high price tag on it, others will learn to save up and buy you at that price.

> **When you value yourself and put a high price tag on it, others will learn to save up and buy you at that price.**

Don't convince others about your worth. First, learn to convince yourself.

GAMES, GAMES, GAMES. STOP PLAYING GAMES.

Test your love. If you're having sex, remove the sex and see if your partner stays loyal or cheats on you. On the flip side, if you're looking to date someone or get into a committed relationship as a virgin or someone practicing purity, bluntly say, "I want to see if you love me, so I want to remove the physical component out of this relationship and focus on connecting with you emotionally and spiritually." If they say yes, don't be happy just yet. We all know that actions speak louder than words.

Many men and women play games, trying to manipulate you out of insecurity from their past or a need for praise and affirmation. You saw that Tiffany and the other women I dated didn't love me for me; rather, they were using me for my looks, my body, my status as a student athlete, or merely for an ego boost, hoping to be the one to say, "I took his V-card, baby! I got him and you ladies didn't." It goes back to that whole flawed concept of the list—the greater your body count, the more worth you have.

Oh, what's that? You're scared to test them? You're comfortable where you are? All right, all right, I gotcha. Let me tell you something: Only when love is put to the test does its real value appear.

Sex can easily become the center of the relationship, dominating over the spiritual and emotional non-negotiable aspects to an authentic, loving relationship. You may not admit that, or you may even not intend it, but if you don't practice self-control and discipline with your passions, you won't be able to get to know your significant other. It's so easy to mistake lust for love, because the world doesn't know what love is anymore. Lust can cover up the absence of true love, being merely a shadow. So what is love? What do you think love is?

You saw how I told Tiffany that I wouldn't sleep with her and she left me in a matter of days. This action immediately showed me what I was being "loved" for. So, if you're looking for a lasting relationship, knowing that you're loved is much more exciting than wondering if you're being used.

I've had a girl tell me, "He promised me sex would make us closer and he was doing it because he wanted to show me he loved me, not because he wanted pleasure. When I stopped having sex, he got mad and left me. I feel like trash. I gave him everything and I was left empty-handed. He wasn't in love with me. He was in love with my body. I wasn't in love with him; I was in love with the feeling of being wanted."

LOOK, IT'S DIRTY OLD LUST

I read somewhere that love waits to give, but lust can't wait to get.

Lust causes a false sense of unity. It's the shadow of love. It appears to be authentic love only to lead to a dead end. It's like the Pokémon Ditto. Ditto can copy into any Pokémon. Although on the outer appearance it seems to be a Snorlax, its inner form is Ditto. You may not see it until it chooses to reveal its true form once it has lured you in. It's also like the pearl analogy. Someone might promise you their pearl, but when you receive it and it rains, you'll realize it was a fake pearl all along. It's hollow on the inside and when the rain washed away the paint, the pearl turned out to be dull, dirty, and lighter in weight.

Giving in to one's hormones which aren't under control and used in the right perspective isn't romance. It's lust disguised as the pearl of love with nothing but hollowness inside. The apple may look shiny on the outside, but when you take a bite, its flesh is poisonous and rotten. You may get sick and even die.

When we experiment with our bodies and souls, we're only training ourselves to value them less and less. You decrease your worth because you keep marketing and selling yourself to people who aren't buying you at full price.

> **The longer you've been practicing purity, the greater your joy and love will be for your future marriage.**

The longer you've been practicing purity, the greater your joy and love will be for your future marriage. I've had people disagree with me on this. I try explaining that it's not my opinion, but the actual truth. Since they can't confront the reality of the truth, they attack it. And yup, you got it—with attacking it comes attacking me. I hear stuff like, "NO! Are you delusional? You should practice in moderation so that you can be prepared for your wedding night," and "You shouldn't be suppressing your desires like that. It's not healthy. It's human nature to have sex. We were born to plant our seeds in more than one person. It's survival of the fittest, man. Get with the game and stop living in 350 BC, ya prude."

I don't blame them. These all sound truthful, but every beautiful lie has a piece of truth to it; that's what makes it so beautiful. But as I said, just like an apple has a shiny outer beauty to it, that doesn't mean it's healthy on the inside. That's why you can have a rotten apple on the inside that's nothing but darkness and poison to your soul.

Are you just going to keep on reading or are you going to take action and test your love? Come on, let me know what ends up happening. I'll be waiting for your response.

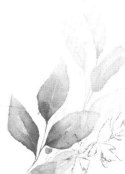

153

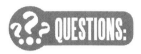 **QUESTIONS:**

1. What's stopping you from testing your love? What are your fears? What social pressures are you facing?
2. Do you find yourself relating to Jeremiah? Why is it so hard for you to wait?
3. What are you really looking for in life? Is sex greater than what you're looking for?

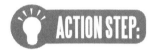 **ACTION STEP:**

1. Make a chart of what lust is and how you can identify it. Now, make a chart of what love is and how you can identify it. Make sure to add the definitions of both. Send me a picture of your answers at coachanthonysimon@gmail.com

19

The Loveable Lies of Love

I hate to break it to ya. . . .
I hate to break it to myself too. . . .
Our truths aren't necessarily the truth.

BEAUTIFUL LIE #1: MY OPINION, FEELINGS, AND MORALS ARE ALWAYS TRUTH

The greatest problem of our time is believing our opinions and feelings are always true, because such a mentality causes us to lose the truth of what makes up a selfless, pure, passionate, flourishing, loving relationship instead of a diminishing, withering, quick-fused, selfish, lustful relationship. What you know to be true is like the colored blob in a lava lamp: It may be real –but only for that moment, and only at your present level of understanding.

This mentality gets you to believe that the only truth that exists is your opinion, so anything that goes against your personal values is seen as a beautiful lie that violates the private world you live in with your own truths disguised as beautiful lies.

A rapist won't get his charges dropped if he argues that in his opinion, according to his value system, raping the child was good and did not violate his personal values. His opinion has no bearing on the fact that some things are objectively wrong. Same goes with a serial killer. The serial killer can say all day long to the cops, "I so strongly felt like that those thirty people in that middle school were planning to kill me. It's not my fault. Please, you have to believe me, I was just doing it in self-defense." You can sit down and try justifying it all you want, but at the end of the day, the truth of the action committed was the person who has a history of being a serial killer murdered thirty people, which is objectively wrong. The evidence of the past and the present point to the person being a manipulative, lost, heartless, killing liar.

If you trust feelings over facts, you'll be used, confused and abused.

The cops and the judge both know that you can't prove feelings. There are actions that point toward feelings, but the facts take precedence over feelings. If you trust feelings over facts, you'll be used, confused and abused. This is why people say actions speak louder than words. Anyone can lie and say "I love you," but at the end of the day, if they don't show you that they love you, then how can you trust them? How do they show you that they love you? This leads to my next beautiful lie.

We can both agree that there are rules to how this world operates. There is a good and a bad. The same goes with love. There are rules to love that, when followed, can help others to flourish, and when they're broken, they cause others to diminish. I like to call these the lovable laws of love, which I discussed in the previous chapter.

It's important to know that how you think and how you feel creates your state of being—physically, intellectually, mentally, emotionally, and spiritually. Most people can't think greater than how they feel, which is why higher principles, standards, laws, and values that should guide our daily choices are removed. Especially in today's generation, this leaves young people with coordinates that only point to their self-absorbed selves and feelings, leading them to the counterfeit of love: lust.

This is why so many relationships fail. The lovable laws of love become an all-you-can-eat buffet, where you pick as much of whatever you want as you want and leave out whatever you don't want. The problem is, people are stubbornly picking unhealthy foods believing they are healthy, out of laziness to do the research, genuinely never knowing, or denial. Everything is based only on feelings, while the mind—the other half of the equation—is being neglected.

> **Everything is based only on feelings, while the mind—the other half of the equation—is being neglected.**

The problem with this mindset is that everyone thinks there is no such thing as right and wrong nowadays. Everyone creates their own moral code based on opinions and feelings rooted in emotions that stem from a bitter past or an uninformed mind and heart. This moral code differs from person to person, and represents a denial of the existence of objective truth. In this mindset, truth becomes whatever you make of it. You hear what you want to hear and you do what you want to do.

You pick and choose only the physical in a relationship, which causes the relationship to burn out quickly because it's only based on pleasure. You're neglecting the emotional and spiritual component of the relationship that are essential for it to flourish.

Living this lifestyle causes a loss of understanding about what's actually a good relationship and what's not. Nobody knows anymore because the truth about love has been covered up by uninformed, misleading opinions. If you seek the truth, you won't be able to find it because there are so many voices polluting the objective truth about what love actually is. These uninformed opinions come from the evil leaders who run this world, looking to decrease your sense of worth and your ability to be loved and love so they can increase in power.

157

LET'S PLAY BASKETBALL

If you play a game of basketball, you'll understand that there are laws the real game of basketball demands: how to dribble, shoot, defend, rebound, pass, sprint, dunk, and steal. If you dribble too far, you might head out of bounds or you may even travel because you didn't know that you can't carry the ball without dribbling it.

Instead of telling basketball how it should be played, basketball tells you how you should play it. Basketball doesn't care about your feelings. The game has already been set in stone and it's your job to find out how to play by researching and putting in the work to become skilled at the game.

The same goes for the game called love. There are rules of how to love and be loved at your fullest capacity that I'll be teaching you. Many fall into the trap of creating the rules to the game of love based on their feelings instead of conforming to the real rules of the game.

Want to know why this is nothing but a comfortable, beautiful lie that's lowering your standards, worth, and ability to love and be loved? It's simple. You're either consciously or subconsciously saying, "It's true for everyone that nothing is true for everyone."

I know. It's deep. So I'm going to put it in another way.

If there is no such thing as truth for everyone, then that is a truth for everyone.

Did you get it? Are you sure? All right, if you say so.

Let's practice. Is this statement true? "There is no truth."

If you answered yes, you are contradicting yourself because if there is no truth, that makes it a truth. Tricky, huh? If you answered no, you understand that this is the same as picking and choosing what you want to believe in or seeing what you want to see and hearing what you want to hear. This mindset becomes a rule whether you realize it or not, which then defeats your opinion that there is no such thing as universal rules.

> *Love needs truth, just as truth needs love. They cannot exist without each other.*

Because of our relativist society, instead

of learning how to recognize and choose right from wrong, you may have been taught how to "clarify your own values." Love needs truth, just as truth needs love. They cannot exist without each other.

When faced with the question "Should I have sex with my girlfriend or boyfriend? Is it the right time to lose my virginity?" you'll look to your feelings only and not the effects of the decision. Instead of asking, "Is this love or lust? Is this right?" you may be asking, "Does this *feel* right? Does this *feel* like love?" This beautiful lie has led countless young people to diminish in their ability to love and be loved because they made destructive decisions based on their feelings that were influenced by their friends, which were influenced by the culture of death—the evil leaders.

It's not about feeling ready; it's about knowing you're ready. This is why we need to grow in wisdom and patience.

BEAUTIFUL LIE #2: PLEASURE IS THE HIGHEST FORM OF JOY

If there is no such thing as right or wrong because there are no rules to the nature of love, why not indulge every pleasure? Right?

Wrong.

People who adopt the mindset of pleasure equals happiness pursue pleasure as their top value, standard, and principle when they should be focused on growth and contribution through disciplining the emotions and purifying their desires through purifying the heart. You may hear them justify it, saying, "It's pointless or impossible to try to control my desires. It's natural. It's the only way to joy." This is the second biggest lie when it comes to relationships. It's a form of denial.

Nobody can live without happiness or pleasure. This is why, when you're not meeting the needs of your soul that leave a *deep* eternal joy; you head to any quick form of pleasure. I'm not saying pleasure is bad—pleasure is instilled in our nature. But if you chase pleasure and happiness, you'll only end more depressed. The more power, status, and sex you get, the more you want. It's a never-ending cycle. That's why we have self-control, one of the virtues you should grow in.

> **Pleasure shouldn't be the main desire in life because it creates an impure heart that demands love instead of requests it.**

Pleasure shouldn't be the main desire in life because it creates an impure heart that demands love instead of requests it. You become selfish and everything becomes about you. Life can't just become about you because it's in our nature to live out our truest desires—growth and contribution. Instead of desiring pleasure, desire what this culture of death calls pain: self-mastery.

Self-mastery is considered unhealthy repression—a borderline mental illness (take it from me, I've been called crazy more than Anthony. Sometimes, I think my name is "Crazy"!)

So what is self-mastery? How do you control your emotions? You master yourself by choosing to wait until marriage to have sex and grow in the purity of your heart through cultivating the virtues of sacrifice, patience, discipline, persistence, courage, and commitment. This increases your delayed gratification and gives you more power. It's why one of my friends who had slept with over fifty women told me, "Anthony, I respect you, man. I wish I had self-control like you. I'm a slave to my desires. How can you go years without porn, sex, or even masturbation? That's just impossible, man. What drives you? How do you do this?"

HOW DO YOU FIGHT THESE BEAUTIFUL LIES?

Relativism and entitlement to pleasure are found everywhere in this culture of death—from the music you listen to, websites on your iPhone, and untruthful sex-ed classes, to the permissiveness of friends' parents. It's possible to break free from the drugs of instant gratification, pleasure, entitlement, and selfishness, but you have to recognize the rules of the game called love.

Both of the beautiful lies I discussed above deny the existence of what's right and wrong and consider waiting until marriage to have sex as a hindrance to personal fulfillment. In today's culture, people risk disease, death, and suffering to gain short-term pleasure. Despite their hearts telling them otherwise, they convince themselves what they are doing isn't wrong by covering up the raw truth with beautiful lies.

The culture used to exalt pure, lasting relationships, but now it exalts the opposite.

The culture used to exalt pure, lasting relationships, but now it exalts the opposite. So how do you fight this? It's easy: You can't. Just give up or go and live on a desert island. The standards nobody wants you to learn are seen as rebellious. And you don't want to be rebellious . . . you want to fit in and give up, even though it means you'll never be loved and love at your fullest capacity.

I'm kidding. I know you want to be loved and love at your fullest capacity.

Don't give up just yet. I'm going to teach you how to escape this self-serving culture of sexual perversion and lead you to the culture of beauty, goodness, and truth. I'll be showing you where to find this culture and how to surround yourself with an atmosphere that is also awake, like you, seeking to get a pure heart by living the same values and standards you have.

You're supposed to live *the* best life of love that leads to *your* best love life. You're supposed to learn the exact blueprint, steps, and motivation to finding the best relationship. The game-changing secrets to finally having the most eternal, deep-set, soul-fulfilling forms of pleasure known to mankind. The catch is, it's going to require effort—which is the exact opposite of what you're used to. Instead of instant gratification, pleasure, entitlement, and selfishness, it's patience, disciplining your emotions and desires, and growing and contributing through selfless sacrifice.

Feeling that someone loves you isn't enough, because what happens when those feelings are gone? Yup, your relationship is gone too. That's why you can't base the foundation of your relationship on feelings only; it must also be with a concrete, logical definition of what love is. A lack of education in the loveable laws of love causes you to rely on your feelings as your only source of truth. Truth becomes truth only if it makes you feel good, but it can't be like that because feelings come and go like the wind and everyone's feelings are different because we all have a different past.

For decades, evil leaders have polluted us with ideas, interpretations, images, and portrayals of sex, relationships, and intimacy that serve to mold what you expect true love to be based on your feelings. They have taken your ability to use your own mind to discover the truth about love. This is why a broad range of people are falling victim to a distorted reality of love, confusing it with lust at every angle. Worst of all, we're surrounded by people who have bought into these beautiful lies that normalize broken relationships, low standards that lead to broken hearts, dysfunctional families, satisfied lifestyles, and deeply suppressed wounds and voids in their hearts. And you're one of them.

Feelings are great, but feelings aren't always truthful, for the heart is deceitful above all things. Your feelings can lead you down a dark path, like they did to me and like they've done to almost everyone in this world at one time or another. You've got to get good at taming your emotions with self-control so that you can dominate them and they don't dominate you.

It's like riding a chariot with horses. Your horses are your emotions. You whip the horses if they are going faster or slower than you desire them to go. You keep whipping them until they learn exactly what you want. You aren't in control of what you feel, but you are in control of how you act. Not everything you feel is true. This is why the universal loveable laws of love have saved so many from relationships where they have failed. They are

Love is a movement of the heart that wills the good of another no matter the pain

concrete truths of what love is and what it isn't. The work has already been done for all of us because relationships always—yes, always—flourish if you follow those rules. If you can take one thing from the loveable laws of love, just know that love is not a feeling; it's an act of the will. Love is a movement of the heart that wills the good of another no matter the pain. Love is selfless and not selfish. Love keeps giving to the point it hurts. How far are you willing to go?

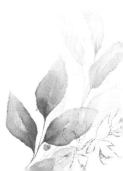

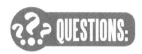 **QUESTIONS:**

1. How have you found that the heart is deceitful above all things in your own life? When have you found it not to be?
2. What does "Love needs truth just as truth needs love" mean to you?
3. When have your feelings led you astray? When has pleasure taken control of your life?

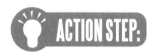 **ACTION STEP:**

1. Look up the terms objective truth, subjective truth, relativism, and hedonism. Now, write down examples of each you found relevant in your own life. I am challenging you to find out where you found your truth or beliefs from. Was it your culture? People? Media? Friends? God? Your Feelings and experiences? Send me your answers at coachanthonysimon@gmail.com

20

The Beautiful Lie: I'm Not Worth Much

I remember I was around five years old when I first experienced rejection. I'm not just talking about any rejection; I'm talking about a deep rejection that altered the way I viewed life. It left multiple scars in the depths of my heart that became the sacred scars I proudly carry today. What's that? How does this story relate to sex, love, and self-worth? Keep reading, and you'll see it come full circle.

In school, it was hard for me to get along with people because I was bullied for having eczema. If you guys know anything about eczema, the more stress you have, the more you scratch. Every morning, I was under constant stress. During elementary school, some classmates and loved ones bullied me and I quickly became labeled as an outcast. There were days I would go to school and try to interact with the girls in my class. They would look at me and say, "Ewwww. Why does your skin look like a crocodile?" Others would say, "Why are your eyelids bleeding? You're gross and weird. Who would ever date you?"

Instead of remaining positive, the darkness entered my mind and I was convinced I was ugly. I was set apart from this world with a heart that just wanted to connect with others. With a heart that just wanted to be asked, "How was your day?" With a heart that wanted to be seen, valued, and cherished. I just wanted to have friends. Was that too much to ask? Was it too much to hear, "Anthony, would you like to play with me?"

I was just a goofy kid who wanted to make people laugh, smile, and feel loved. But the world said no. I was bullied for even trying.

ARE PEOPLE'S WORDS STEALING YOUR JOY?

You see, I was born a positive kid who was surrounded by negative people. Think of a little puppy finally freed from his cage, trying to run around and play while sniffing other puppies. It didn't help that I also was socially awkward, underweight, and very slow in school. I'd go to school and people made fun of me because I was small, didn't get good grades, and would cry because I didn't understand how to read or write. I couldn't focus in school because I was such a free, creative thinker who was a lot slower and more anxious than everyone else. I did not like following the rules or sitting down and taking standardized tests. I was an outsider—an alien monkey living among civilized human beings.

I still remember the day I cheated off the smartest kid in our class. The question said, "Write the number 5," so I drew it with five dots and then looked at my classmate's paper and saw I was completely wrong. The teacher noticed I was cheating and eventually, the whole class found out because I cried in front of everyone. A classmate and his brother said, "Hahaha! You're stupid. You can't read or write. Dummy. I'm smart and you're dumb."

I remember defending myself, saying, "At least I can play basketball."

They replied, "What are you talking about? You're a toothpick. You're not athletic and you're short. You're not good at basketball. I saw you play. You're not good at anything. You're useless."

You're smart if you're asking, "How can you still remember something that happened at that young of an age? It was kindergarten and elementary school dude." Well, it just goes to show you how much that affected me.

What I still don't believe is how I was battling negativity while I was so young. It's not usual for a kid to be severely bullied like I was. Kids don't know how to react to pain at that young of an age; their brains are still adjusting. This causes trauma and alters the brain of a child. The needs of my soul weren't being met. I was told I was illiterate. I was told I couldn't read or write well. I was told I was anxious about speaking in public. I was told I was stupid. I was told I was worthless. I was told I was ugly. I was told I was worth nothing. I was told I had no value. I was told nobody would ever find me attractive.

HAVE PEOPLE'S OPINIONS OF YOU SHAPED YOUR REALITY?

I became very insecure at such a young age and suffered from public speaking anxiety. When people would call me out to read in class, I would freeze or not know where they left off. My insecurities, anxiety, and lack of focus were so bad the teachers placed me in special education. I was told to my face, "Are you stupid? ANOTHER F!?!?!?! You're such a failure! You're wasting your parents' money." Some said, "You're never going to amount to anything. Are you even trying?" Many teasingly said, "Do you even speak English?" Others told me, "Why aren't you like your brothers? They are all straight-A students. You're useless. Why do you exist?"

But there was hope! Things started to pick up when I became the center of attention. What attention and how did they pick up? Well, the pain only got worse and I got attention all right—attention as the class punching bag and clown. The pain snowballed and I became the target to be made fun of, bullied, used, backstabbed, ignored, rejected, isolated, laughed at, not acknowledged, and even given fake attention and love just to get whatever my classmates wanted.

There were many lunches I sat alone eating in the corners of the playground. I was an outcast. I felt homeless, yet I had a home. All I wanted was a friend. All I wanted was to hear the words, "I'm proud of you. You're a good man. I love you." All I wanted was unconditional

167

love, not conditional love based on my performance in the classroom, my looks, or my athletic abilities. All I wanted was to be myself instead of hiding behind a dark mask.

All I wanted was to know I had a purpose. Did I have any meaning? Did I have any value or worth? Did I have a future? Why was I alive? Why was it worth living life?

The only friend I had was my dark mind. My inner demons were the only people I knew. I'd go home to a stressful environment because I wasn't the golden child living up to my family and relatives expectations. I lived in the shadows of my brothers, who were praised for doing well in school. I was nothing but a failure who got Fs, Ds and even 23 percent on his homework and tests. I still remember flushing those grades down the toilet to hide them from my parents. I still remember people laughing in my face saying, "What did you get? OH, DANG! Thirty-three percent! AHAHAHA! I've never met anyone that dumb in my life. Did you even try?" They didn't know what I was going through.

I was told to my face, "Why are you wasting your life dribbling a basketball? You're never going to make it. You're a failure and will always be one. Give up." The saddest part was this wasn't only my classmates, teachers, and relatives; this was also my family . . . my only source of love left. I thought family was supposed to support and love each other, not tear each other down. Because of these experiences as well as others I cannot mention out of respect, I had a twisted understanding of what love was. I was in deep pain with no source of love in my life. I didn't feel accepted by anyone, not even my own self.

WANDERING FOR WORTH

I often questioned, "Why do I have to suffer so much? Why can't I find love? Does love even exist? What is and isn't love? If love exists, where can I find love? Is there really a plan for me or am I destined to be a failure like everyone says? Why am I so different from everyone else? Why do I feel like the black sheep in the family? Why am I not like my brothers, cousins, and family members? Am I adopted?" I searched for answers to these questions, but as a child, you can only know so much.

I couldn't find any answers so my anger turned to depression. I became hopeless. I remember closing the door in my closet and sobbing like it was my last day. I was afraid of the dark, yet I still chose to head straight toward my fears. I stayed there for hours crying, saying:

"I NEED HELP! Is there anyone out there for me? PLEASE!"

I dreaded going to school many days. At times, I wanted to skip school because I couldn't handle the pressure and the pain. I just wanted to be loved. I just wanted to be seen. Was there anyone out there to love me? Where could I get love? I was thirsting and hungering for love. I allowed others to tell me my worth because I didn't understand my worth.

SEXY SACRED SCARS

I bring this childhood story up because we all have hidden wounds waiting to be healed. We all have non-negotiable needs of our soul: respect, trust, connection, feeling valued/cherished, physical touch, intimacy, and community. If you didn't hear words like "I love you" or "I'm proud of you" in your childhood, chances are you were neglected as a kid and you're seeking that affirmation in others, especially relationships.

> *We suppress these wounds by getting into relationships looking for affirmation and healing through others when we should be first looking within ourselves.*

Many of us carry these unseen and hidden traumas that drive us to seek to bandage these wounds with outside sources of love. We suppress these wounds by getting into relationships looking for affirmation and healing through others when we should be first looking within ourselves. We're waiting for that attention and love we never got as children from our family members.

These hidden traumas are in all of us. I call them hidden because most of us aren't aware of the needs of the soul and body because we've always been deprived of them. I mean, even a monkey can see that our newer generations are struggling more and more with depression, anxiety, loneliness, heartbreak, insecurities, and mental illnesses.

These wounds only get worse because most of us don't pay close attention to our feelings and thoughts. Instead, we numb them with short-lived pleasures not only because it's painful to confront these issues, but also because we don't know where to start. We have no guidance and never truly meet the deep desires of our soul. Healing comes from exposing beautiful lies. Healing comes from identifying, embracing, and working toward solving them, no matter how painful they may be. I was fortunate enough to be healed from my dark past, and now I hope to be that guide for you, too.

> **Part of being human is that you and I both have a past where we've been wounded.**

Part of being human is that you and I both have a past where we've been wounded. Nobody has perfect parents; some of you may only have had one parent, some none. You don't live in a perfect world—you're bound to get hurt. It's inevitable to avoid relationship hardships: painful heartbreaks, failed marriages, abusive relationships, manipulative boyfriends, controlling or seducing girlfriends, neglect, loneliness, mental illness, trauma, fathers or mothers leaving you, or even parents who didn't have enough time to hang out with you or give healthy amounts of physical contact. Part of getting hurt means you get the joy of having a past that haunts you for the rest of your life . . . or does it have to be that way? Can you actually be freed from your past and let go of it?

Many bitter people will lie to you, saying, "You have to deal with the reality of the situation. You can't be fully healed. You'll always be heartbroken. You might as well give up already. I don't know anyone who has survived. You'll always have scars for the rest of your life; there's no way around it."

I like to respond with, "Who said my scars can't be sacred scars?" It is possible to let your greatest relationship *tragedies* turn into your greatest relationship *treasures*. It's not only possible to completely heal from your scars, but it's also even completely possible to erase all the haunting memories from the past. If you think you're inadequate because you lost your virginity or because you still have it, think again. It doesn't matter if you are or aren't a virgin. What matters is the purity of your heart and mind. The past is the past and your current situation isn't the end of your chapter. What matters is the desire to change and heal and learn from your past, and the willingness to do it.

TRANSFORM TRAUMA TO TREASURES

Listen.

Statistics said I was never going to find true love. Statistics said I was never going to graduate college, let alone high school. Statistics said I would be depressed my whole life. Statistics said I shouldn't even be alive right now, but by some miraculous grace and mercy, I'm alive. I was granted the opportunity to be here to serve you now and this is why I'll never give up on you. I shouldn't be here right now but I am, and for that, I desire from the depths of my soul to help heal you and bring you the joy that I have, too. I overcame my greatest traumas and transformed them to my greatest treasures.

You may be currently chained up by horrific, screeching, rusty, heavy, smelly chains that have been weighing your heart and your spirit down. You may be fighting your inner demons only to listen to their comforting, beautiful lie that whispers, "It's okay. Life is supposed to be this way. Just accept and embrace it and move on. You'll find love eventually. Just keep doing what you're doing." You may have spent years searching and finally finding the key to unlock those gruesome chains, only to find out you don't know where the lock even is. Heck, maybe you can't even figure out how to unlock the chain even though you have the key in your right hand. So, you give up and

> *It's no wonder so many of us believe love isn't possible. We have yet to heal our wounds from the past.*

suppress the pain deep in your heart thinking one day it will go away. After all, you can't show emotions because the culture tells you not too, right? Wrong.

It's no wonder so many of us believe love isn't possible. We have yet to heal our wounds from the past. We keep telling ourselves the same story: "I was neglected as a child. I'm not worth much because I have such a dark past. I was cheated on; therefore, there's something wrong with me. I'm not worth much because people don't love or believe in me. Since I was rejected at home or rejected by my previous relationship, I'm not good enough. I'm only as good as I am accepted and loved by others. They define who I am."

I don't know anything about your past, nor do I know how painful it was, but I do know one thing for certain:

Pain is pain. It falls on the good and the bad. It's not about our troubles being different. Our pains are quite similar, even though they may stem from different events and be of different degrees; it's our solutions that are different.

How you handle the pain with the right perspective, as I talk about in my best-selling book, *Life's Greatest Gift: P.A.I.N.,* will dictate how you grow through it and not just go through it. Before you give up searching for love, you should know true love exists. Draw your hope from knowing I'm not the only one who was freed from my dark chains and past. There are many people out there that have followed the same path and are still being loved and loving at their fullest potential.

You've got to take it from the most insecure kid who has ever walked in this planet: Love is real. It does exist. The beginning of your journey doesn't start when you make the decision to start; rather, the journey starts when you have given everything you got and put your hands on your face, crying, saying, "I give up!" That's when your search for love begins. That's when you realize that just because this is a chapter of your life, doesn't mean it's your whole story. You may be on Chapter 20 (see what I did there?) but you still have more chapters to finish reading to see how your story ends.

When you can realize that your worst days are truly your best days and that every human being goes through unfair pain (some more than others), then you've taken the first step. Everyone has had someone who they trusted or loved and cared for deeply hurt them. Everyone has had someone who they've looked to for support and love be unjust to them. It's part of how we grow spiritual muscles.

Think of it like lifting. There's no possibility to build strong muscles without lifting heavy weights. If you don't lift the bar, it will crush you, but if you lift it, it will be painful. Just like weights, it's not easy lifting those problems, but the day you finally find insight within your inner self is the day you're no longer pressed down by your past. That's the day your life not only changes but you learn how to receive, build, and give the same gift of love to others. This is your worth. You'll find yourself saying, "If it wasn't for all that I hated most, I wouldn't have what I loved most. Growing in the purity of my heart made me realize that there's a meaning greater than just serving little old me."

THIS IS JUST A SEASON

Most people think the temporary pains are the permanent things. The temporary passing pain of going through a breakup. The temporary passing pain of getting cheated on. The temporary passing pain of being rejected as a kid by your own family. The temporary passing pain of despair. You don't understand that you're going to be okay if you fight and try healing from those wounds. When you're in a low and feeling bad, you think how you're feeling is how you're going to feel forever, which is what makes it feel worse.

Part of letting go is healing. Your past does not define you. It does not determine your worth.

All of your emotions are temporary. I keep saying it: feelings come and go like the wind. They're passing things. So, most of our pain stems from believing that we should keep holding onto these things that are really heavy in our lives.

Learn to let go of the past.

Part of letting go is healing. Your past does not define you. It does not determine your worth. Don't listen to the world telling you you're not good enough because of what happened to you. Who are they to tell you your worth? Why do you listen to them? What gives their opinions validity? You have to learn how to extract the good from the bad of what they say, but how do you do that? How do you know what is actually the truth and what isn't?

We're so afraid of being vulnerable, real, and honest because we're terrified of being judged and held to a standard that society sets for us. Decide that you're worth more and take action by finding out who you are. The only way you're going to get strength in your life is by healing from that tough moment.

Your belief is what sustains the wound. If you continue to believe that you aren't worthy of love, you're not good enough, or you allow your past to chain you and define your worth, you're never going to heal. The belief that we get our worth based on the love of others isn't true. Don't listen to these dark thoughts because they control our feelings and our feelings control our actions. We end up wasting our lives constantly comparing rather than repairing these wounds.

This is why so many of us suffer deeply from insecurities. Our insecurities manifest through drugs, alcohol, sex, goals, achievements, popularity, power, and attention. All of these insecurities and forms of restlessness try and fill the void of love in our heart. Even though we all have different ways of coping with our dark past to fill the rejected and wounded pieces of our hearts, we all have one need in common: the need for affirmation from others. Affirmations point to our greatest desire and need—to be fully seen for our authentic selves and to love and be loved fully.

You may have had a dark past that wounded you deeply. Instead of healing those wounds by accepting the truth they point to, you're quick to listen to the world telling you, "Deny. Run away." You may have chosen to cover them up with comfortable, beautiful lies by going to the world searching for love when you should've spent time building yourself and understanding what it means to love and be loved fully first. In this case, you have already sold your pearl, but if you confront your fears, you can gain your pearl.

Are you ready to confront your greatest fears to be made perfect in love?

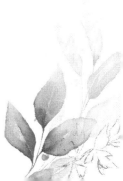

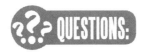 **QUESTIONS:**

1. What is your dark past? Think all the way back to when you were a kid. Were you rejected and unloved? How did that make you feel? What did that cause you to do? Were there moments of your life when you didn't feel good enough?
2. Did you hear "I love you" or "I'm proud of you" or "You're handsome/beautiful?"
3. What "drugs" are you taking to numb your pain?

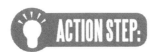 **ACTION STEP:**

1. Write down every painful experience from your past. Confront everyone who has hurt you in your life. Write it down and learn to let go, embrace it and forgive no more how painful it may have been. Feel free to share with me at coachanthonysimon@gmail.com

21
Wandering for Worth

'd had enough.

I wanted to be seen.

I wanted to be valued.

I wanted to be known.

I wanted someone to recognize my talents, gifts, and charisms.

I wanted people to finally see me the way I saw my authentic self.

I wanted a consistent source of love. Not just any love. Unconditional love.

I knew there was no medicine or quick fix-it-all pill that would cure my emotional pain and fill the void in my hardened heart. I began to discover that true poverty wasn't just people out in the streets, it was lack of love in one's life.

I constantly played the story back in my mind. "You're not good enough. You will never find love. You're ugly. You need to get bigger, stronger, manlier, smarter, charming, smoother, and funnier. You're not enough, little boy. The love you talk about doesn't exist. Stop living in a fantasy world, kiddo. Just give up. Why even try? You should just end it all and join everyone else. You should've given those women your virginity. Stop living a pure life in mind, body, and soul. The only way these women will stay with you is if you give it all up."

I kept hearing the narrative in my head. "Women aren't worth your time. You shouldn't be committed to just one when you can get more than one. Become a man. Get your power back. All your friends and teammates are doing it. Start chasing as many women as you can—that's what's going to fill this void in your heart. You hear me? These women don't want to be respected—they're nothing but trashy girls who want sex. So, treat them like trash."

This voice just came out of nowhere. It sounded so truthful and really hit home on all my wounds. It continued, telling me everything I wanted to hear. "It's not settling; it's called growing up. You're too old-fashioned. Nobody cares to wait until marriage anymore. Those people don't exist. It's just you. So why don't you just join the trend of the world and make your pain go away? You have a lot of women who are waiting for you, Anthony. Aren't they pretty? You still have two more years left to experiment in college. That's plenty of time to have fun and gain experience. Go to parties and see what's out there before it's too late. I mean, if you really want to have a good marriage, you should test-drive the car before you buy it. You should learn how to be good at sex now so you can impress your wife later. You haven't even had your first kiss yet. You're such a child. GROW UP! BE A MAN! CLAIM YOUR MANHOOD BACK! NOW IS YOUR TIME!"

I was tired of giving pieces of my heart to people who didn't deserve it.

I was tired of getting cheated on. I was tired of the fleeting relationships. I was tired of not being valued. I was tired of holding on to my standards. I was tired of giving pieces of my heart to people who didn't deserve it. I was tired. I was tired of hiding behind a mask. I was tired of giving more, expecting to receive more and not receiving a thing. I was tired.

Being cheated on, emotionally rejected, denied, isolated, abandoned, abused, and bullied only made me suffer. I lost my self-esteem, my value, and my worth. I was born in darkness and being hardened by pain. I was surrounded by everyone who seemed so loved and I was sitting in the darkness.

I kept getting used and manipulated for striving to be the "nice guy." I would build myself back up and try again only to get let down. After trusting and giving the benefit of the doubt, I was let down. If you've ever broken through your walls of doubt and fear and let someone in only to be deceived, you know exactly what I'm talking about. It's hard to trust others again, let alone trust yourself.

I just wanted to be loved. I wanted to be loved DEEPLY! I was THIRSTING for love. I was STARVING without love. I didn't have the greatest upbringing. I suffered from emotional, mental, and verbal abuse. Rejection and loneliness was most of what I experienced as a kid. I wondered why I was going through so much pain as a kid. Life didn't make sense to me.

I started asking questions like, "Who am I? What am I on this planet to do? Am I delusional? Am I crazy? Where is my identity?" I was losing control and I wanted to gain that power back. I wanted to feel strong again. I wanted to feel like a man, so I decided it was time to make a change. It was time to crush hearts.

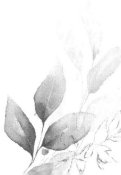

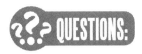 **QUESTIONS:**

1. Where do you draw your worth from? Where do you draw your identity from?
2. When have you heard a similar voice like mine in your life saying, "Give up. Lower your standards"? Did you listen? Did you resist? Why?
3. How have your wounds from family or previous relationships affected you?

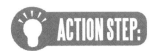 **ACTION STEP:**

1. Write down everything that makes up your identity. Now, rank them in order. Why are they in that order? Feel free to share with me at coachanthonysimon@gmail.com

22

I'm Sorry. Please Forgive Me

I'm sorry.
I'm sorry with all my heart.

I'm sorry to all the women that I have manipulated, hurt, left feeling emptier, played games with, and made more lost. I'm sorry to all the women I treated as objects instead of human beings. I'm sorry for using words to smooth-talk my way to your heart only to steal what's not mine and crush it to stroke my own ego. Please forgive me.

I'm sorry to all the men out there for not having the courage or strength to stand up for my vision and acting like a player. I'm sorry for being a boy and not a man. I'm sorry with all my heart. Please forgive me.

I was thinking with my body and not with my brain, trying to hide my scars by looking for some quick pleasure to lessen the burden in my heart. I can tell you that the time you spend chasing women or men actually works against you and your desire to improve yourself in mind, body, and spirit. It only makes you more depressed, lost, and wounded. Don't listen to the world that says otherwise. It's all a lie. It's not worth fitting in. It's not worth lying to yourself and saying you're in love when you're clearly being used. It's not worth feeling accepted for a couple of minutes only to be quickly reduced to a piece of meat. It's not worth it.

I misunderstood my desire to be loved, interpreting it as the desire to show others how "smooth" or "charming" I was by turning girl's heads and not hearts with my body, words, or actions. I craved to be seen. I craved to be valued. I craved to be the center of attention. In the eyes of my "friends," I was the player who had muscles, a six-pack, the reputation, and game. I gave them the impression that I would have sex with a ton of women and that I was the "alpha" when in reality I was just a vain virgin boy who had never even kissed a girl.

The chase and the games become like a drug addict chasing the next high.

The chase and the games become like a drug addict chasing the next high. At first it's fabulous, but then the high only has a lower and lower affect and you find yourself becoming a slave. You want to break free because it pains you, but you can't stop. Having a physical or emotional connection feels great in the beginning. You love the thrill of the chase. Playing the games keeps you up on your toes and the unknown of whether or not they like you back is thrilling. It's not so thrilling when you ride the downs of the roller coaster, though. How do you feel when you've bene reduced to nothing but a piece of meat or ghosted, rejected, judged, or even manipulated?

As silly as this sounds right now, I was the one doing the ghosting, manipulating, judging, and rejecting. Welcome to the majority of my life in college. I'm not going to sit here and lie to you—I was a very vain, broken, insecure boy breaking hearts and leading others to believe I was someone I wasn't for attention.

How did all this start? What led me here? I think it's time to share this part of my story.

THE ONE WORD NOBODY LIKES TO SAY

Pornography.

Pornography affected my view on sex, my worth, and love by

leaving me more insecure, leading me to use people to fill the void in my heart and my insecurities.

Believe it or not, I found myself stumbling across pornography and masturbation at around six years old. I found out about it in school and quickly became addicted because it temporarily met the needs of my soul—the same needs I wasn't receiving as a kid.

I know. Six years old. How is that even possible? I don't know.

All I knew was that extreme pain called for desperate measures. I was living in darkness. Everywhere I looked there was darkness. Some may call this depression; I called it hell on earth. I wanted to be loved, but I wasn't loved. I wanted to be seen, but I wasn't seen. I wanted to be heard, but I wasn't heard.

Darkness. Darkness all around me.

Who would've ever known a kid that young can become plagued by his inner demons of depression, insecurity, anxiety, worthlessness, anger, and isolation? How was I forming soul ties with a computer screen at such a young age? The scariest part was I became conditioned to this lifestyle. I thought this was life—darkness written the rest of my days. I can't sit here and lie to you. I thought life was only suffering and I was hopeless to change.

I was in darkness—deep, thick, blinding, soul-eating darkness. I hated myself. I wanted to escape but I couldn't. I was a deeply wounded kid who resorted to pornography and masturbation to heal his wounds.

As I got older, my medicine dosage of pornography and masturbation only increased. As my medicine increased, the purity of my heart decreased and I began to objectify women and treat them trashier with each video I watched. At the time I felt like I needed the drugs. This was the only fix I knew, even if it was only a temporary one. I needed to get the needs of my soul met. I needed to find my worth by reducing women to my playthings and breaking their hearts. This is what pornography taught me. This addiction

Even though it takes only a few seconds to see the pictures, it takes years to forget them.

to porn and masturbation stayed with me all the way until nineteen years old. Finally, at nineteen, I found the cure.

Pornography at such a young age rewired the chemistry in my brain and trained me to see the value of a woman based on how much I lusted over her. How much she could initially attract me with her hotness and body was how much I pursued. Even though it takes only a few seconds to see the pictures, it takes years to forget them. Pornography taught me to reduce others to sexual objects that can be used and then discarded once my passion wore off and the emotions left. It taught me to play with hearts and reject the responsibility of being with a woman.

Remember the chemicals I was talking about in Section I? You are forming a bond with pornography when you watch it and the consequence is an inability to connect or bond with a real person in front of you. You saw it happen with me. I couldn't connect with women because I connected with porn. I know I dated a lot of immoral girls, but I also dated several moral girls whom I still wasn't able to connect with. No matter how good the woman was, I still would say something was wrong with them when, in fact, I was the problem. Finding love became a game of breaking hearts instead of building hearts.

You also saw this with Hugh Hefner, the founder of Playboy's multi-billion-dollar porn empire. Hugh had access to the most desirable and sought-after women, but he had to have pornographic material in the bedroom for him to reach any stimulation. His brain has been so bonded with hyper-performed sexualized images that a real flesh-and-blood person was not enough.[1]

Unrealistic expectations and fantasy ideals surface when you think you'll be able to perform at the same level as porn.

Unrealistic expectations and fantasy ideals surface when you think you'll be able to perform at the same level as porn. You may say they're only actors or models, but your hormones don't know that. You can bond internally to specific images, ideas, and fantasies to the point where "normal" sex with your spouse isn't exciting anymore.

When you do this, you rob yourself of the true intimacy, connection, and comfort that you were created for.

I'M NOT THE ONLY ONE

Think it's just my experience? I'm not the only one. Listen to what these husbands, wives, and couples said about the negative effects of porn and premarital sex:

"I divorced my husband because he loved porn more than me. I caught him watching porn in our room several times. I always told him to stop and he told me he would but he never did. It got to the point where I just rolled my eyes because I knew he'd never change and I would always be used. I couldn't feel loved by him anymore so I decided to divorce him as I became an object to him."

"Living under the fantasies, unrealistic expectations, and illusions of porn destroyed my marriage. I'm divorced because I couldn't learn to love my wife. For many years I tried but couldn't get those images out of my brain and she knew by the way I acted in the bedroom. It killed my marriage, man. Killed it."

"Listen, man, porn sets the standards for your spouse to live up to a fantasy and provide as much excitement. Porn and hookups trained my brain to associate sex with dirty sexual fantasies of countless disposable women. It's unrealistic, which is why my spouse felt insecure. You don't mean to make them feel that way but you can't control getting rid of these thoughts and unrealistic expectations. You become conditioned."

One couple said, "Porn caused those distortions of our sexual desires . . . we struggled against in order to discover true love. Masturbation achieves neither bonding or babies. Instead of communicating life and love, you're only selfishly satisfying your own needs with yourself through lust."

Another couple said, "Sex before marriage becomes 'me' instead of 'we.' It becomes 'How much can I get instead of how much can I give?' We both became objects of lust, not objects of love."

You see, nobody will talk about these things because they live in fear of the opinions of other people. They don't want to be judged so they hide under a rock and close their eyes and live with the mentality of, "If I can't see you, you can't see me." This flawed logic is completely torn apart. We can all see it by the way you live your life. You don't have to tell us because your actions are already speaking for themselves. True strength is admitting you're weak and taking massive action.

> **Everyone always acts like everything is okay on the outside but in reality they are hiding all of their darkness.**

Everyone always acts like everything is okay on the outside but in reality they are hiding all of their darkness. They try and suppress it with temporary fixes of pleasure that only create a bigger void and darkness in their heart. I would head to parties to get attention from women. I was so brokenhearted that I used to play games and manipulate women so I could stroke my ego and get validation that I was good-looking. My insecurities and addictions took control of my life. Worst of all, I judged women and would say, "My lifestyle is justifiable because I'm still a virgin. That makes me a clean person." I failed to realize that I was lusting after women, creating soul ties without even knowing it, and most surprisingly, avoiding some of the deepest wounds that I didn't know existed in my life.

VAIN VIRGINITY VOW

I had the wrong equation of love. I didn't know what it was and I was seeking but couldn't find it. I wanted to be a man, but I was only a boy thinking he was a man. The world would tell me what it meant to be a *man* but I felt like a *boy* who was never happy. I'd be happy for an instant because of the attention and approval I got from people's opinions, but it would only temporarily fix the problem, leaving me feeling worse in the end.

I was HUNGRY for finding love. I was STARVING and THIRSTING.

I mean, there were some days I was thinking about ending it all because I didn't get the love. I hated my life and I was being controlled by my desires of lust, physical intimacy, emotional and spiritual intimacy, pornography, masturbation, and stealing women's hearts.

I was a slave convincing myself I was free. But if I truly were free, why would I feel so ashamed on the inside? Why did I lack so much self-worth? Why did I have a terrible relationship with others, especially the women in front of me? Why wasn't I able to focus? How could I focus? What was freedom? What did it feel like to be free?

I had no focus and lost all my energy. I wasn't motivated to accomplish any of my goals and I was one of the most insecure people you would've ever found on the planet. I was fully dead and became so depressed that I wanted to take my own life away. Had I not had any faith or hope I would've done so. It was terrible and I felt like throwing up some days because I wanted to escape but didn't know how. There were some days where I couldn't get out of bed because of how wounded I was living this lifestyle.

But no. I had to act like everything was perfect on the outside. I had to put that mask on thinking I was free. You see, what I learned from my mistakes is that true freedom isn't the ability to do whatever you want. True freedom is doing what's right even if that means taking the hardest path that nobody else dares to take. True freedom is the ability to set higher standards instead of lowering them. Holding firmer to the vision instead of having no vision. Controlling your desires instead of being controlled by them. Living life fully alive instead of fully dead. True freedom is what you're doing now—seeking to get into an intimate relationship to find authentic love.

I don't know what you may have felt. Your story may be similar to mine or completely different. But I do know that we share one truth in common: We're both looking for stable, consistent, unconditional love to heal our wounds—love that we can draw near to our broken hearts and crushed spirits. We can relate because we have the same non-negotiable human needs of the soul. It's in our DNA.

I began to understand that, like everyone else, I was searching for something . . . something I had no idea where to find.

I began to finally sit down and use my brain for once. I started to journal and asked myself, "What is love? Pure, selfless love?" If you're reading this book, you're looking for more. Well, what is it that "more" you're looking for?

What are you looking for in your life? What desires in your heart are demanding your attention? Have you finally fulfilled these desires or have you become a slave to their never-ending demands? Is what you have enough for you or are you looking for more?

I finally found out what I wanted: a constant source of love. I was placing my identity in women, basketball, my achievements, my family, my values, my virtues and standards, my worth, and my relationships, but none of these were consistent, perfect forms of love that were stable. I didn't want to base my worth on others and their affirmations and opinions. I wanted to base it on the truth about who I am.

So I finally had discovered what it was I was looking for. The only question was, what is the truth about me? Who am I? What is my purpose? What am I going to do with my life? Despite my mistakes and failures I shared with you in this chapter, I was still empty, restless, and thirsty for love.

I questioned myself. I desired change. I desired to love fully and be loved fully.

I started to ask, "What is love?" I didn't think my definition was right. I wondered where I got my definition of love in the first place. When did I first learn about it? Why is it that when I'm dating someone and they tell me they love me, I don't feel it? Why do they show me they love me yet I don't feel it? There had to be some sort of beautiful lie either they or I was believing about love.

It wasn't until I desired love more than I desired pain that I not only made the conscious decision to change, but also put an effort to seek authentic, lasting love. It was then I realized that in order to give and receive love at its fullest capacity, I had to understand what love actually was and wasn't.

It wasn't that I was looking for things in the wrong place; I was simply looking for them in the places where I demanded they be found. The very last bit of my self-esteem was crushed because I decided to let my identity and worth come from the opinions of others at a deeper level.

I started to ask my inner self if I should go back to my vision. "Should I keep loving my future wife? Does authentic love exist? Is love real? And if it is, is love still worth fighting for despite being so empty and causing so much hurt? Should I take my walls back down?"

Love? Love? LOVE? Where are you?

Inner self? Inner self? INNER SELF? WHERE ARE YOU?

Please. Please. Please, just show yourself.

Show yourself just this one time before it's too late.

I. Need. Help.

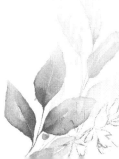

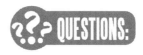 **QUESTIONS:**

1. When have you caught yourself saying, "I need help?" What did you do during those times?
2. Are you a slave to pornography and masturbation? How has it affected your relationships?
3. When did you catch yourself lowering your standards in life? How is that related to your self-esteem? How can you increase your self-esteem?

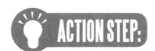 **ACTION STEP:**

1. If you struggle with sex before marriage, shallow hook ups, porn or masturbation, write down all the harm, shame, insecurity, lack of focus and destruction it has caused in your life. Write down the triggers too. Why are you doing them? Finally write down how it is destroying your vision of love. Now, make a plan of action to stop. Feel free to share with me at coachanthonysimon@gmail.com

PART 3
Building Love
& Worth

23

A Love Letter From Love Itself

Inner Self: I heard your cry for love. I heard your pleading. Listen, I know you're in pain. It's time for you to read the letter from the king's son. I draw near to the broken-hearted and the crushed in spirit.

You: Yeah, man, I'm really having a hard time trying to find myself. This may be my last sense of hope before I decide to give up and quit on finding love.

Inner Self: I know. I'm sorry I've had to wait this long but you weren't ready. Now is the time. I've been waiting for you. Now read!

THE GREATEST STORY EVER TOLD

Among us, there once lived a son sent by a king
He was the king's son, no ordinary human being
He was our hero
Despite the world seeing him as zero

The king saw the brokenness in our relationship
And decided it was time to deliver us from the slave ship

The king felt our pain with compassion
He knew his son was the only one who could take action
So he took a chance and rolled the dice
He sent his son to the world and made the sacrifice

Knowing his only son would die, the king knew what he had to do
He loved his son, how could his tears not be so blue?
His father sent him to take all the pain
So we could potentially live with all the gain
His father loved him but knew he had to pay the price
Because we were so lost, his father made the sacrifice

His son had a vision to restore love
His mission captured people's eyes like a tender dove
He said, "Rich or poor well it doesn't matter.
Weak or strong, you know love is what we're after.
We're all broken, so pay attention to my words spoken."

The world hated him because of envy
He indeed restored love; being called people's excellency
With his story, he took the world's glory

He was the light in our world of darkness
He put up a fight for those so heartless
Not knowing love, we were lost thinking we're found
Our relationships suffered but he turned that all around

We lived in beautiful lies thinking we could see
But we had yet to know the truth that could set us free
None of us understood the truth about love at the time
But now we clearly see, proclaiming, "I'm ready to shine!"

He washed our mistakes clean, as white as snow
With mercy and grace, none of us would ever know

With many stripes, he took the loss
He swallowed death and he paid the cost
He took the time to get us right
He gave us all he had. He gave his life

Worst of all, besides his great fall
The world wanted nothing to do with him at all
At one point, you and I hated him too
But while we were killing him, he forgave us, saying, "You know not what you do."

You: Why do you sound so familiar? Where have I heard this poem before? It's like it's written in my heart. Who are you?

Inner Self: Who do you think I am?

You: Uhhh. . . . Yeah, man . . . that's why I'm asking you.

Inner Self: . . . .

You: Hellooooooooo?

Inner Self: . . . .

You: DUDE! Why do you always disappear like that the moment I'm about to hit a breakthrough?

Inner Self: . . . .

You: Oh, let me guess . . . you want me to think about it. You're sooooo annoying but I kind of like it at the same time. Fine, fine, fine. I'll give it some thought. See ya in the next chapter of my own life.

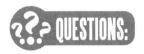

QUESTIONS:

1. What did you learn from this story?
2. Were there any times in your life you were thirsting for love but didn't know where or how to get it? What did you do?
3. Who do you think the inner self is? Why?

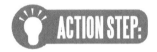

ACTION STEP:

1. Highlight and write down what parts of this story hit your heart hard. Write down why they touched your heart. Email me your answers at coachanthonysimon@gmail.com

24
Be Satisfied With Me

Inner Self: So, who do you say that I am?

You: I . . . I . . . I still don't know.

Inner Self: Do you remember that one person you dated?

You: Who? Oh . . . wait . . . wait a minute. I remember.

Inner Self: Remember the note they told you to read?

You: Yeah, but I don't know where it is.

Inner Self: Check your right pocket.

You: What the?!?!?! Dude. How do you keep doing this?

Inner Self: I can't give away my secrets. Don't worry about it. Just read for now.

BE SATISFIED WITH ME

Everyone longs to give themselves completely to someone,
To have a deep soul relationship with another,
To be loved thoroughly and exclusively.

But I say, "No, not until you are satisfied,
Fulfilled and content with being loved by me alone.
With giving yourself totally and unreservedly to me.
With having an intensely personal and unique relationship with me alone.

When you discover that only in me is your satisfaction to be found,
You will be capable of the perfect human relationship,
That I have planned for you.
You will never be united to another
Until you are united with Me.
Exclusive of anyone or anything else.
Exclusive of any other desires or longings.
I want you to stop planning, to stop wishing, and allow me to give you
The most thrilling plan that exists . . . one you cannot imagine.
I want you to have the best. Please allow Me to bring it to you.

You just keep watching me, expecting the greatest things.
Keep experiencing the satisfaction that I am.
Keep listening and learning the things that I tell you.
Just wait, that's all. Don't be anxious, don't worry,
Don't look around at things others have gotten
Or that I have given them.
Don't look around at the things you think you want,
Just keep looking off and away up to me,
Or you'll miss what I want to show you.
And then, when you're ready. I'll surprise you with a love
Far more wonderful than you could dream of.

You see, until you are ready, and until the one I have for you is ready,
I am working even at this moment
To have both of you ready at the same time.
Until you are both satisfied exclusively with me
And the life I prepared for you,
You won't be able to experience the love that exemplifies your relationships with me.
And this is perfect love.

And dear one, I want you to have this most wonderful love;
I want you to see in the flesh a picture of your relationships with me.
And to enjoy materially and concretely the everlasting union of beauty, perfection and
Love that I offer you with myself.
Know that I love you utterly. I am God. Believe it and be satisfied with me.

I AM

You: God. . . ?

God: I am. I am agape. I am unconditional love. I am in you. I am the creator of the loveable laws of love for I am love itself. I am the love that you are longing for. I am the secret to every successful marriage and relationship. To fully love another and have a successful relationship, you must first learn to draw from the well of living water and living love—Me. I am the one who can restore your relationships, heal your wounds, and show you how to receive love to give love. I am the light who will set you free from your darkness. I am the source of life. I am the way. I am the truth. I am the life. I am the love. I am the joy. I am not *a way, a truth, a life, a love, a life, a joy* . . . I am *the way, the truth, the life, the love, the life, and the joy* that you desire. It's a bold claim I make. Either I'm a liar, a lunatic, or indeed your Lord. Test Me.

You: I've always heard of You but there are just so many people that talk about You, and they say a lot of different things. How do I know who to believe? How do I know who to trust? Everyone claims to say they know You, but who are You?

God: There are so many who know Me but they don't have a relationship with Me. They continue to make relationships with others, never knowing what it means to love because they have yet to find Me. It's simple: Find Me. Find yourself. Find your relationship. I want to bless these people with the best relationship but how can I do so when they aren't ready? How can I bless them if it's going to cause them more pain in the long run because both of them still have yet to understand what it means to live in unconditional love? It's impossible to do so without Me. I'm that hidden secret magic potion in the love lab.

You: So . . . wait. Just wait a minute. Anthony has been talking about you and your teachings this whole time?

God: Ta-da! I knew you would catch on. Everything you learned about sex, love and your worth is the truth because I am the truth for I am love. Remember chapter 4? I am the pearl. I am your worth. I am your key. I am your map. Those are My words you were reading. You can trust them because I am God and I want the best for you. I am the source of all truth. Remember Chapter 6? The Loveable Laws of Love you've learned originated from Me. Remember Chapter 9? I made the chemicals in your brain so that they can attach and bond to only one person—your spouse. Love comes from me. Everyone who loves knows Me.

I AM WHO YOU'RE LOOKING FOR

God: So, you may ask, if I am love and love is in you, then why don't you feel loved sometimes? It's because you have yet to get to know Me and My power within you. There are natural rules I operate in your world.

If you can get to know Me more, you'll find out the answers to all your questions about your identity and life itself. I'll let you know about your worth and if you're that 128-ounce cup waiting to be filled with My love or that 32-ounce cup. Let Me tell you everything about you. Let Me tell you how precious you are. How much you're worth. How much I believe in you. How much I want you to succeed. Let Me show you the most transcendent love life you can get. Let Me show you that I am your God—the one deepest desire you're looking for.

You: How do I get there? What do I do?

God: You have yet to take Me out on a date. You may say you believe in Me, but it's not enough to believe in Me, for even My enemies believe in Me and know who I am. My enemies know all the words about who I am too. It's not just enough to know Me. You must have a relationship with Me. My whole life I've been chasing you. I chose you, you did not choose Me. I don't want anything but your heart. I want all of you but I'm afraid you don't want all of Me. That's okay; I still chase you hoping that one day, just one day, you can experience the joy I have for you.

You: But . . . but what do you want from me?

God: I want nothing more but for you to be happy every day of your life. I want to reveal your identity through Me. I want to reveal why you're in this earth. I want nothing more but to heal your wounds so you can have a loyal, loving marriage with not only your spouse, but Me too. I want nothing more but to restore your purity with a new pure heart and a new pure mind. I want nothing more than to be the father you never had or never felt loved by. I want nothing more but to see you have the best marriage of your life so that you can understand how much I love you through the sacrament of marriage.

You: I feel like you've been so distant my whole life. I'm just so lost. You say you're love but I don't feel it.

God: Every relationship is a two-way street. You've been talking to Me your whole life, telling Me what's wrong, what you want from Me, making demands, and not requests. You've been treating Me like Santa Claus. Even though you're on My naughty list for turning against Me and breaking our covenant together, I still give you what you desire even though you don't deserve it, you hurt My feelings, and you haven't done anything to earn it. You treat My mercy so casually. My graces are available for you to receive every day but you never ask Me for them. You never say sorry and you get mad at Me, blaming Me for your pain when you could've avoided it if you just said hello to me every now and then. What hurts Me the most is that you fail to realize what I do for you. I don't know how many times you've spit on Me, made fun of Me, backstabbed Me, and cursed on Me when I continue to bless you with gifts in your life. The problem is, you don't see these as gifts since you always expect them to come. I don't owe you anything since you choose to be with Me only when things go bad. You just expect Me to give you whatever your heart desires when it's not always what will make you the happiest.

I AM DESPERATE FOR YOUR LOVE

You: Dang. I'm sorry. I didn't know, God. Please forgive me.

God: I do. I just want you to know that it hurts Me because you never take the time to listen to what I have to say. You know, I have emotions too. Sometimes I cry. Sometimes I get mad. Sometimes I am heartbroken. You are My creation, but I want you to be My child and live as My child, free from all lies and all darkness. That's why when you do come, I'm quick to love you and listen to what you have to say. I'm quick to show you comforting signs to let you know that I am your God and remind you of My promises.

You: What are your promises?

God: Can you please just listen to what I have to tell you for once? I want to teach you My promises. I want to teach you how to be happy. I didn't make rules, teachings, and guidelines to follow to punish, manipulate, or restrict you. I made instructions on how to live your life happily, free of worry, and in perfect love. All you need to do is listen to what I have to say. Can you do that for Me? You can have such a better life than the one you're living right now. I am the healing that you're looking for. I am the desires hidden within your heart. I am that satisfaction that nothing else can give you. I promise you so much. So, so much. Just take My hand and allow Me to lead you. Do you believe? Do you trust in Me?

You: I just. . . . I'm just scared. I'm scared of the unknown. I don't want to lose my control. I'm selfish. I want to do what I want to do. There are so many different philosophies about you that I just get more lost, restless, confused, and discouraged. Every time I put in the effort to get to know you, I don't see any progress. I feel like your words are lies because they never come true. I don't see them applying in my life. If I just stick to my morals, I should be all good and avoid hell. I'll still get to heaven, but what even is heaven? Oh, great, angels singing, the tree of life, and apples. I don't really feel that motivated; I'm comfortable the way I'm living now.

God: Comfortable? You were not made for comfort. You were made for greatness. I'm trying to take you to another dimension. What do you want out of life? What are your deepest desires?

You: I just want to be happy. I want perfect happiness. I want perfect justice. I want perfect truth. I want perfect love. I want to be a hero. I want to love. I want to make a difference in this world. I want to make a difference with my family. I want to grow and I want to contribute. I want to leave a legacy.

God: I promise all those and more, but I want you to understand this: It's not just about getting to heaven. You're missing the point. You're going to die one day. One day, you're going to meet with Me face to face and I'm going to ask you, "Why should you get to heaven? What have you done?" What would you say?

You: Well, I don't know. I'd say proudly that I raised a family. I was a good person. I lived the morals I thought were best. I loved my neighbor and I . . . uhm . . . I don't know . . . I didn't do anything bad. I went to a couple churches here and there. I mean, like, isn't that what life is? Living your best life according to the morals you were given and just being a nice person overall?

God: I'll tell you that those are all good things with the right intention but I'll look you in the eyes and say, "There was more and that wasn't enough." I intended for you to be the greatest creation I ever made, but because you let fear, doubt, lack of trust in Me, selfishness, pride, and wanting to control and be your own creator stop you, you didn't make the cut. You refused to listen to what I had to tell you, no matter how many times I tried to warn you that you were going on the wrong path and were being led by the enemy. I kept chasing you, sending you signs and opportunities to change, saying, "Look out! Don't go there. It's a trap. It looks good, but it's just a mirage until the prison door slams shut. You won't be able to leave. Please, listen to Me. I know all things. I see all things. Don't do it." You refused to listen and because I created you with free will, I didn't want to take it away. It hurt Me deeply, but I didn't give up on you. I gave you one final chance at the last hour of your death, but you just couldn't forgive those couple of people who hurt you. Why would you expect Me to forgive you? Why do you deserve to sit with Me when you never wanted to? How would that make you feel?

You: I . . . I . . . I don't know what to say. That's just so deep for me. What do I do to get to heaven? What even is heaven? Why should I care?

God: Heaven is full intimacy and oneness with Me. It's a fulfillment of all the desires of your heart. It's total peace, joy, love happiness, truth, and beauty. Heaven is your true home. I created you to be in full communion with me. The laws are written in your heart and consciousness. All you need to do is trust Me. Trust Me. I love you and I'm proud of you for continuing to talk with Me. You've got such a bright future ahead of you. You have yet to discover what can happen to you when you take My hand and allow you to guide you. Your future spouse is waiting for you, but you first must take My hand.

You: What do I do to take Your hand? How do I follow you?

God: I need to heal the wounds in your soul. I need to teach you about My love so you know what to look for in your future spouse.

You: How are you going to do that? I don't even know where to start.

God: I made everything easy for you. Here. Read the last section on giving love and worth. All you need to do is read the love letter that I have made for you. These are My exact words and through them, you'll find out more about Me and how precious I've created you to be.

You: I just. . . . I just hope it's all worth it. This may be the very last time I give You a chance.

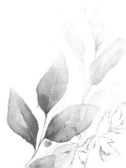

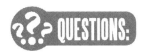 **QUESTIONS:**

1. What struck you in this chapter? What questions do you have about God? Doubts? Fears?
2. If today were your last day, what dreams would die with you? Would you die with regret?
3. Do you desire to have a relationship with God to learn to love others better and find out your truest worth? What can you do to get there? What's the next step?

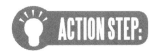 **ACTION STEP:**

1. If you're ready, pray this prayer to God. "God, I don't know who you are nor do I know if you're even real. Can you please shower your love and joy on me? I want to be happy but I just don't know what to do. Can you direct my steps?" Now, write down all your wounds you need healing from. If you're not ready, write down any questions you have about God. Write down how you view God and why you view him that way. I want to hear your questions and experiences. Email me at coachanthonysimon@ gmail.com and we'll talk about them.

PART 4
Giving Love & Worth

25

Love Revealed

Dear Precious Child,

GOD, WHAT DO YOU WANT FROM ME?

You're probably asking right now, what do I want from you? Let Me tell you. I came to give you life and life abundantly through unconditional love. I want you to live life to the fullest (John 10:10). I want to meet all your needs (Philippians 4:19) and bless you abundantly, so that in all things at all times, you will have all that you need and will flourish in every good work (2 Corinthians 9:8). I want you to take delight in Me so I can give you all the desires of your heart and ones you don't even know about (Psalm 37:4). I want to fill you with eternal pleasures and joy in My presence (Psalm 16:11).

Don't believe Me? Test Me in this and see if I will not throw open the floodgates of heaven and pour out so much blessing that there will not be room enough to store it (Malachi 3:10). If you trust in Me, I will give you what you desire and make all your plans succeed (Psalm 20:4). Just trust Me and My promises and I'll make known to you the path of life (Psalm 16:11). I want to give you more than what you ask for or imagine. Just trust Me and allow Me to equip you with everything good for doing My will by working in you. Want to know My greatest secret? When you trust Me, you're content in any and every situation (Philippians 4:12). As you trust Me, you allow My power to work within you (Ephesians 3:20). You will then know that I am the God of hope who will fill you with all joy and peace so that you may overflow with hope. When you trust Me, My power works within you and you understand that you can do all things through Me who strengthens you (Philippians 4:13). When you trust Me, it pleases Me, for I desire to save you by having you come to full knowledge of the truth about love (1 Timothy 2:3-4). All I ask is that you love Me back and all My blessings will be upon you (Exodus 23:25).

Do you love Me? Do you trust in Me?

DO I REALLY LOVE YOU?

I know there are so many people who don't believe in My love for them. That's because they never listen to what I have to say through My words. Let Me tell you how much I love you. Write these words down, for this is nothing but the truth and they will make you a new creation (Revelations 21:5).

If you could just grasp how wide and long and high and deep is the love I have for you. If you could just know this love surpasses all knowledge (Ephesians 3:18-19), you'd know that I have loved you with an everlasting love; I have drawn you with unfailing kindness (Jeremiah 31:3). You are precious and honorable in My sight. Why? Because I love you (Isaiah 43:3). Don't believe Me? Indeed, the very hairs of your head are all numbered. Don't be afraid; you are worth more than many sparrows (Luke 12:7). You are fearfully and wonderfully made. Your works are wonderful; I know that very well about you (Psalm 139:14). How do I know this about you? I have searched you and I know you. I know when you sit and when you rise. I see your thoughts before you think them (Psalm 139:1-2). Before I formed you in the womb, I knew you and called you by name. Before you were born I set you apart and appointed you to speak about My love for you to all nations (Jeremiah 1:5). I formed your inward parts; I knitted you together in your mother's womb (Psalm 139:13).

Most importantly, My child, this is how I showed my love among you: I sent My one and only Son to the world that you might live through him. This is love: not that you loved Me, but that I loved you and sent My Son as an atoning sacrifice for your sins (John 4:9-10). I so loved the world that I gave My only Son, that whoever believes in Him shall not perish but have eternal life (John 3:16). Very rarely will anyone die for a righteous person, though for a good person someone might possibly dare to die. But I showed My love for you and everyone in that while you were all still sinners, I sent My only Son to die for everyone (Romans 5:7-9). My Son, Jesus Christ, died for everyone's sins, was buried, and raised on the third day (1 Corinthians 15:3-4). He took all the pain and bore your sufferings, stricken and afflicted by every sin committed. I was wounded for your transgressions; I was crushed for your sin, injustice, and wrongdoing. The punishments required for your wellbeing fell on Me, and by My wounds, you are healed (Isaiah 53:4-5). Even though My Son was crucified on the cross because of your sins, My Son still said to Me, "Father, forgive them, for they do not know what they are doing" (Luke 23:34).

As I have loved My son, Jesus, so I have loved you (John 15:9). Dear friend, since I so loved you, you also ought to love one another. If you love one another, I live in you and My love is made complete in you (John 4:11-12).

Do you trust in Me?

GOD, I FEEL BROKENHEARTED AND CRUSHED IN SPIRIT

If you're feeling brokenhearted, know that I heal the brokenhearted and bind up their wounds (Psalm 147:3). To proclaim freedom to you, the captive, I bind your broken heart and release you, the prisoner, from your darkness (Isaiah 61:1). I hear your cries and will deliver you from all your troubles. I am close to the brokenhearted and save those who are crushed in spirit. I will protect all your bones and not one of them will be broken. No one who stays within My covenant will be hurt (Psalm 34:17-22). Just ask Me to create in you a clean heart and renew a right spirit within you. Ask Me to always stay close to My heart and near Me through the Holy Spirit (Psalm 51:10). I want you to look unto Me and continue waiting for Me, your God of salvation. I will hear you. When you fall say, "I shall arise"; when you sit in darkness, I shall be a light unto you (Micah 7:7-8). One day you will say, "I called to the Lord, who is worthy of praise, and I have been saved from My enemies" (Psalm 18:3). You will then know that I am forgiving and good, abounding in love to all who call upon Me (Psalm 86:5).

FORGET YOU, GOD. I DON'T NEED YOU

Please, don't give up on Me. Don't insist on your own ways. I want you—all of you. I don't want 80 percent of your heart. No . . . not even 99 percent of your heart. I want 120 percent of your heart. I say 120 percent because I am God and I will always give you more than what is humanly possible. You see, until you can learn to give Me your 100 percent, you will never experience the life I designed for you to have. There is nobody like you, which is why I'll keep relentlessly chasing you until your deathbed. When I breathed life into you, I gave you My image and likeness. I gave you a piece of Me. I want you back. Please, My heart is incomplete with you, My dear child. The same loneliness you have is only a fraction of what I am feeling that I am not fully with you because I don't have your full heart.

I will chase you like a dog chasing a car. Even though the dog may not catch the car, the dog is just hoping that the car will stop at a stop sign or a stop light so it can get your attention. I am that dog. I want you to stop. Stop pressing on the gas and allow Me to show you that I thirst for you like a dog thirsts for water after chasing you for so many years.

Allow Me to meet you face-to-face and you'll see My thirsting, joyful eyes. Allow yourself to return to Me like an owner who has returned to their dog who was tied on a leash to a tree for the whole day. I've been waiting for not just days, but years. Not knowing when you'll come back, I still waited for you patiently and loyally, believing that maybe just one day you would come back into My loving, embracing arms.

Do you feel My pain? Do you feel My love now? All you have to do is return to Me, My child. Please, come back. How much longer should I wait? You are My child and I'm waiting for you to return home (Luke 15:11-32).

Do you trust in Me to continue reading My love letter? I have so much more I want to tell you, but first I want you to read about how Anthony even found Me.

Your Loving Father,
God

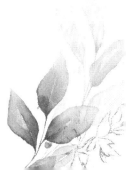

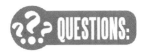

QUESTIONS:

1. What questions do you have about God? Are you going to give Him your heart? How will you do this?
2. How can you get these questions answered? Do you even care about Him?
3. Why do you think it's important to care about God and actually follow Him?

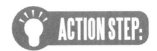

ACTION STEP:

1. Ask God to reveal Himself to you and give you a sign of His love. Now, write down all the times you've felt loved by God. Write down what God has done for you in your own personal life. Also, remember the list of all your wounds? Bring them to God and ask Him to heal you. Share your responses with me coachanthonysimon@gmail.com

26

December 8, 2017

It happened on December 8, 2017, at around 7 p.m. My life would never be the same again—never.

God had been chasing me my whole life, trying to teach me the fullness of love and how much I was worth. Despite yelling at God, blaming Him, calling Him and His words nothing but manipulative lies, and intentionally going against His teachings and commandments in His church and the Bible, He continued to chase me. The more I ran away, the more brokenhearted I was, and the more crushed in spirit I was, the closer God came into my life. Despite all of my bitterness, anger, and resentment toward God for feeling abandoned, He spared my life several times while I was going through a dark night of my own soul.

That fact that I am alive today is a miracle in itself. Sitting here having the undeserved privilege to write this book is a miracle that I never anticipated in my life. God transformed me from being a brokenhearted man who was crushed in spirit and fully dead to a fully alive, energetic, joyful person. He was able to turn my scars to sacred scars. He turned my greatest tragedies to my greatest testimonies. Statistics say I was supposed to be dead multiple times in my life, but God allowed me to understand who He was on December 8, 2017. Before I tell you what actually happened on that day, I want you to see the love letter He helped me piece together to get a clearer picture of who He actually is.

GOD'S LOVE LETTER CONTINUED

My Precious Child,

So, it looks like you trusted Me enough to continue reading My love letter. I love you so much and am so proud of you. For many years, Anthony cried to Me from the depths of his soul. During these dark times in his life, he felt as if I had abandoned him because he thought his prayers weren't being answered. If you're wondering why your prayers aren't being answered, if My promises aren't true, why you're feeling abandoned, or even how to build a relationship with Me, read the same love note I revealed to Anthony. Look how happy Anthony is now because of the light I shed in his life. I want to do the same for you.

YOUR PROMISES DON'T SEEM TRUE!
I FEEL LIKE YOU'RE LYING

Know this: I never lie and My promises are always true (Titus 1:2). I am not slow in keeping My promises as you understand "slow" (2 Peter 3:9). Just because My promises don't come to pass on your time doesn't mean they aren't true. Submit to Me just as a patient with cancer submits to the surgeon. I am your creator and My time isn't your time (John 7:6).

You must understand that just as light exists, darkness does too (John 1:5). The devil and his demons are very real and they are thieves that come only to steal, kill, and destroy the blessings I am trying to give you. By using doubts, fears, and lies, they cause you to distrust My promises (John 10:10). Once you lose trust, you lose My blessings because you fall under despair, lack of peace, conflicts, anxiety, depression, and many more weapons of the devil.

The devil is very cunning. Just as Eve was deceived by the devil's cunning lies, your minds may somehow be led astray from your sincere and pure devotion to me and My words (2 Corinthians 11:3). So I want you to write My words down for they are nothing but the truth (Revelations 21:5). The devil will try and pluck My words out of your minds (Mark 4:1-20), but be assured that My light shines in the darkness, and the darkness has not overcome My light. I have already won the battle. Just rely on Me and My strength and not your own efforts (John 1:5).

Don't allow Satan to fill your heart with lies and cause you to lie against My promises (Acts 5:3). Test every voice you hear (1 John 4:1-6), for even your own heart, feelings, and emotions are deceitful above all things (Jeremiah 17:9).

GOD, DID YOU ABANDON ME? I AM IN DARKNESS

You must remember My promises. You have forgotten My promises. Do not forget My promises. Always meditate on them (Psalm 103:2). Again, everything works in My time (Ecclesiastes 3) for My ways and thoughts are not your ways and thoughts (Isaiah 55:8-9). You'll be superbly happy if you trust in Me and have confidence in My words, for when I deliver you in My time, I will over-deliver and flood your heart with unexplainable joy.

My son, pay attention to what I say: turn your ear to My words. Do not let them out of your sight; keep them within your heart, for they are life to those who find them and health to one's whole body (Proverbs 4:20-22). My words are a lamp unto your feet and a light unto your path (Psalm 119:105). If you hold to My words and teachings, then you will know the truth and the truth will set you free from the darkness (John 8:31-32).

By My words I have created you (Genesis 1:26) so use them to combat the lies of the devil, for life and death are in the power of the tongue and whatever you speak, you'll eat its fruit (Proverbs 18:21). For My words are not chained (2 Timothy 2:8); My words are living and powerful, and sharper than any two-edged sword, piercing even to the division of soul and spirit, and joints and marrow, and act as a discerner of the thoughts and intents of your heart (Hebrews 4:12). Reflect on what I am saying, for I will give you insight into all this (2 Timothy 2:7).

I will fight for you; you need only to be still and trust in My timing (Exodus 14:14), for if I am within you, you will not fall. You shall not be moved. I shall help you (Psalm 46:5). I Myself will go before you and will be with you; I will never leave you nor forsake you. Do not be afraid; do not be discouraged (Deuteronomy 31:8). I give strength to the weary and increase the power of the weak (Isaiah 40:29).

Can a mother forget the baby at her breast and have no compassion for the child she has borne? Though she may forget, I will not forget you! See, I have engraved you on the palms of My hands; your walls are ever before Me (Isaiah 49:15-16).

Cry out to Me in trouble and I will save you from your distress. I will bring you out of the utter darkness and break away your chains. All you need to do is remain in My unfailing love and give thanks for the wonderful deeds I'm doing for you (Psalm 107:13-16). Your sun will never set again, and your moon will wane no more; I will be your everlasting light, and your days of sorrow will end (Isaiah 60:20).

Also know that abandonment is the result of your sins and rebellion against Me and the wrong choices of other human beings (Genesis 3). My own chosen people suffered and felt abandoned when they disobeyed My covenant by breaking My commandments (Deuteronomy 28). I allow you to feel abandoned so you may understand the consequences of sin and turn to Me and repent so that you won't perish for eternity (Luke 13:1-4).

If you listen carefully to Me and do what is right in My eyes, if you pay attention to My commands and live out all My teachings, you will be protected (Exodus 15:26). Then you will call on Me and come and pray to Me, and I will listen to you. You will seek Me and find Me when you seek Me with all your heart. I will be found by you and I'll bring you back from captivity (Jeremiah 29:12-14).

WHY AREN'T MY PRAYERS BEING ANSWERED THEN?

If you aren't already seeking Me and trying to build a relationship with Me, then how do you expect Me to answer your prayers? I'm trying to teach you to seek Me while I may be found and to call on Me while I am near (Isaiah 55:6). When you seek Me, you live. If you do not seek Me, you are not remaining in Me, but if you remain in Me and My words remain in you, ask whatever you wish, and it will be done for you. If it's not done, it wasn't according to My will and I have something better in store for you that you don't see now. Trust Me (John 15:7). So, do not worry about anything, for I know what you need before you even know what you need (Matthew 6:31-32). Which of you fathers, if your son asks for a fish, will give him a snake instead? Trust that I am your perfect loving Father. I will not give you what will ruin your life. Trust Me (Luke 11:11).

Maybe you do not receive because you do not ask Me. When you ask, you do not receive, because you ask with wrong, selfish motives, that you may spend what you get on your pleasures (James 4:2-3). You do not receive because I have made everything beautiful in its time. Nobody can fathom what I have done from beginning to end, for I have set eternity in the human heart (Ecclesiastes 3:11).

If you, My creation, who are called by My name, will humble yourself and pray and seek My face and turn from your wicked ways, then I will hear from heaven, and I will forgive your sin and will indeed heal you. Now My eyes will be open and My ears attentive to your prayers offered (2 Chronicles 7:14-15). I listen to Godly people who do My will (John 9:31).

GOD, HOW DO I BUILD A RELATIONSHIP WITH YOU?

So how do you actually build a relationship with Me? Before I teach you how to restore your relationship with Me, you must first build it. To build a relationship with Me, there are specific rules you have to follow (2 Timothy 2:5).

Rule #1: I am your God whom you should earnestly seek. Your whole being should thirst and long for Me knowing that I am your help and you should cling to Me. I desire that you love Me not only with your words but actions too (Psalm 63:1). When you seek Me, you live (Amos 5:4). If you seek first heaven and a relationship with Me, everything will be given to you (Matthew 6:33). You need to make the most of every opportunity by seeking My will (Ephesians 5:16-17). If you lack wisdom about what My will is for your life, ask Me and it'll be given to you (James 1:5).

Here I am! I stand at your door and knock. If anyone hears My voice and opens the door, I will come in and eat with that person, and they with Me. I wait until you're ready and that's why the teacher doesn't show up until the student is ready to learn (Revelations 3:20). I am your teacher who looks down from heaven on all mankind to see if there is anyone who understands Me, anyone who seeks Me, anyone who is ready to learn (Psalm 53:2). Whoever has ears, let them hear (Matthew 11:15), for My sheep hear My voice, and I know them, and they follow Me to eternal life (John 10:27-28).

Rule #2: I want to establish a covenant with you—a special relationship with you—one making you a new creation, born again as My child (John 3:3-4). You will become My sons and daughters when you receive the sacrament of baptism and confirmation, since the same spirit that exists in Me will be in your hearts. You can then call Me Father! (Galatians 4:6). I will be in you forever through the Holy Spirit, who is another helper and the spirit of truth. He will dwell in you and be in you (John 14:16-17). The Holy Spirit is your comforter and supporter whom I sent in My name. He will teach, reveal, and bring to memory everything I need you to know and do. Through the baptism of the Holy Spirit, I will direct your heart (2 Thessalonians 3:5). You won't be able to enter heaven or build a relationship with Me unless you are baptized with water and spirit! (John 3:5). When you are baptized, you are given new birth into a living hope through the resurrection of Jesus Christ from the dead, and into an inheritance saved in heaven for you that can never perish, spoil, or fade (1 Peter 1:3-4). Lastly, if you are My child through baptism, My Son, Jesus Christ, will live in you, protecting you from the enemy. Jesus is greater than the devil who is in the world (1 John 4:4).

Rule #3: Learn to love me back.

HOW DO I LOVE YOU?

It's very simple. If you love Me, keep My commands. (John 14:15) As I have loved My Son, Jesus, so I have loved you. Now, remain in My love. If you keep My commands, you will remain in My love, just as My son has kept My commands and remained in My love. (John 15:9) What is My command? My command is this: Love each other as I have loved you. There is no greater love than this: to lay down one's life for one's friends. You are My friends if you do what I ask. I tell you this so that My joy may be in you and that your joy may be complete (John 15:11-17). This is how love is made complete among you (1 John 4:16-17).

Remember My ten commandments? My first five commandments can be summed into this: You shall love Me with all your heart and with all your soul and with all your mind (Matthew 22:37). Also, you shall love Me with all your strength and with all your body (Deuteronomy 6:5). My last five commandments can be summed into this: Love your neighbor as yourself (Mark 12:31). Follow Anthony's action step at the end of this chapter to learn more.

Now I know you may be asking, "What is love?" You can have faith to move mountains, but if you do not have love, you are nothing. If you give all you possess to the poor but do not have love, you gain nothing. Love is patient. Love is kind. It does not envy, it does not boast, and it is not proud. It does not dishonor others, it is not self-seeking, it is not easily angered, and it keeps no record of wrongs. Love does not delight in evil but rejoices with the truth. It always protects, always trusts, always hopes, and always perseveres. Love never fails (1 Corinthians 13).

My love never fails. Will you allow Me to love you? Will you trust Me?

HOW DO I RESTORE MY RELATIONSHIP WITH YOU?

So you've made a couple mistakes. Okay, I get it. You're only human. You may have not followed My commandments but now you feel like trying. That's right where I want you. Listen up, My child.

When you sin, you cut relationship with Me and then belong to the devil because you carry out his will and desires (John 8:44). You must learn how to purify your heart and desires by asking for My mercy and graces through the sacrament of confession. You will be superbly happy if you have a pure heart because you will see Me (Matthew 5:8). If you do not purify your heart, your desires will give birth to sin, and sin, when it is fully grown, brings forth death (James 1:14-15). Walk in the Holy Spirit through baptism and you shall not fulfill the lust of your flesh (Galatians 5:16-17), for I will be in you fighting against the sin and providing the escape route. I will not let you be tempted beyond what you can bear (1 Corinthians 10:13).

If you confess your sins, I am faithful and just and will forgive your sins and purify you from all unrighteousness (1 John 1:9). Allow Me to wash away and cleanse your sins as white as snow (Isaiah 1:18), for I am compassionate, gracious, slow to anger, and abounding in love. I will not always accuse, nor harbor My anger forever. I do not treat you according to your sins or ask you to repay Me for sinning. For as high as the heavens are above the earth, so great is My love for you if you truly love and seek Me. As far as the east is from the west, so far have I removed your sins from our relationship (Psalm 1038-12). Just make sure to be sorry from the bottom of your heart. Make a full act of contrition for the wrong you have done (Numbers 5:7). If you acknowledge you sin to Me and not cover up your iniquities, I will forgive the guilt of your sins (Psalm 32:5).

When you become aware that what you're doing is a sin, you are guilty and need to truly be sorry for your sin (Leviticus 5:5). In this case, do not conceal your sins, otherwise you will not prosper, but confess and renounce them and you will find My mercy (Proverbs 28:13). When you do this, know that My tender mercy will come from heaven like the rising sun (Luke 1:78) and I will forgive your wickedness and will remember your sins no more (Hebrews 8:12). For I am very patient with you, not wanting you to perish but to come to repentance (2 Peter 3:9).

I am light and in Me there is no darkness. You must walk in My light by purifying yourself from all sin to be one with Me. The blood of My Son, Jesus, purifies you from all your sins; you need only to confess your sins. If you claim to be without sin, you deceive yourself and the truth is not in you (1 John 1:5-10).

WHAT ACTUALLY HAPPENED TO ANTHONY ON DECEMBER 8, 2017

Let Me take you back to the long, lonely, devastating nights I had with Anthony. For many years, Anthony was so lost in thick, blinding, darkness because of the lifestyle he was living. He neglected Me many times and prioritized his own ways above Mine because he wanted to be the creator of his own life. By consciously and knowingly living in sin without putting forth an effort to change, he had cut off his relationship with Me. I sent him so many signs and opportunities to change his ways but he refused to. He kept telling Me to go away and leave his life, so one day I decided to answer that prayer.

Anthony was My precious baby and I didn't want to see him suffer, but because of his free will, I honored his decision to live the life that he wanted. What he didn't know was that it pained Me to see him suffer more than it pained him, but this was the life that he chose.

His free will to disown Me caused him to drift away from My sight, breaking our covenant. He didn't repent for his sins from the bottom of his heart, so it didn't restore our covenant, making him a slave to the devil. Anthony became the devil's stringed puppet, and this made him feel lost, abandoned, unloved, rejected, despised, and even unheard by Me.

For years, Anthony lived on the strings of the devil. When immense pain began to settle into his soul, Anthony began to realize that he wanted Me back in his life. There were many nights he cried for hours begging Me to spare him from the darkness he was enduring. Anthony cried to Me and for every tear he shed, I had shed hundreds more, for I felt his sorrow very deeply. He always asked me, If you're all loving and powerful, why am I suffering? Little did he know, he would turn his 1033 pages of journaling and reflecting to a book answering that question.

Listen to his words he prayed to Me every night as he cried in the same chapel while firmly grasping a statue of the Blessed Virgin Mary and a picture of My Son, Jesus Christ. Anthony said, "Mom, Mom. I wanna go home. Please, I can't take this anymore. I asked you to be my Mother, your Son Jesus to be my Brother, and God to be my Father when I was five and a half years old. Mom, I don't feel Dad's presence anymore. I feel as if God has abandoned me. Mom, where is Jesus? I've been crying to Him for years, just like I'm doing to You right now, and He only increases my pain. Where is He? I can't, Mom. I can't go on anymore. This is it. You're my last hope. I have reached my lowest point. Mom, do you hear me? Mom, does my broken heart lie? Help. Help Me. HELP! God! Where are you, God? Hear my cry, Lord."

As he began pleading and calling for help from the depths of his soul with every ounce of pain, his tears began rushing down his cheeks and I was moved to compassion hearing his prayer. He thought I wasn't hearing him so I sent him the Holy Spirit, which brought electrifying goosebumps surging from his head to his toes for a long duration that made him feel understood, heard, and comforted by Me.

He continued talking to the Blessed Virgin Mary, saying, "Your baby is hurt. Can you please spare me? Mom, dad (God) isn't listening and my Brother (Jesus Christ) isn't listening to my prayers either. You're my last hope. Please. Please. Please save me from this darkness. Deliver me from this darkness. Heal me from this darkness. Mom, don't forget about me. I feel forgotten. I feel abandoned. I feel as if I don't have a heart anymore. Please. I can't take it anymore. I need your help. Tell Dad I'll do whatever He wants. Tell your son Jesus I'll win Him souls for the kingdom of God. I love You, Mom, you're the only one left who will understand me. I heard you hear the cry of your baby children in a more tender way than Jesus. Please, hear my cry. Feel my pain. Convince your Son to spare my soul and fill my heart with His grace and mercy."

Although he didn't know it at the time, his prayers truly moved Me with compassion toward him, but I couldn't just take him back so quickly. I wanted him to understand the consequences of sin and know that I truly want what's best for him. I wasn't going to save him until he could learn the lessons I was trying to communicate to him through his pain. Even though Anthony was unrighteous with Me, I felt his pain, for he never gave up on Me and never gave up seeking the lessons I was trying to communicate with him.

Finally, on December 8, 2017, I was convinced by the Blessed Virgin Mary to spare Anthony's soul. She had taken his prayers to My throne in place of him and offered them up to Me as red roses. She had convinced Me why I should spare him sooner because of his devotion to Her. In that moment I decided to spare Anthony's cold, bitter, hardened heart and calloused mind that was consumed by darkness. On that day, I told the Blessed Virgin Mary that She had permission to lift the veil of darkness blinding him.

If you didn't know, December 8 is the date of the Immaculate Conception, which is the birth of the Blessed Virgin Mary. It's no coincidence that I sent the Blessed Virgin Mary to grab Anthony and lead him to My Son, Jesus Christ, on that day. Even though Anthony was still a slave to his sins, I had mercy on him by sending the Blessed Virgin Mary.

With My permission, the Blessed Virgin Mary went to work on his life and instructed Anthony on how to become one with Me by building and restoring our relationship. Through supernatural experiences and accompanying signs, she helped Anthony piece together that all along, my Son, Jesus Christ, had been chasing him, trying to teach him how to finally find love by first finding Me. She taught him that I am a real, breathing, living, all-powerful, all-knowing, loving father who wants the best for him by living in the fullness of truth, fullness of justice, fullness of beauty, and fullness of love.

He received the sacrament anointing of the sick, as well as special blessings from priests, which helped him attend adoration frequently, read the Bible consistently, and receive my graces and mercies through the sacraments of Eucharistic Communion and Reconciliation. He began exponentially growing and life finally clicked for him. He understood what it meant to have a relationship with Me first and it went from his mind to My heart through confession, frequent Eucharistic communion, reading my words, and frequent Eucharistic adoration.

Although he still has much work to do and he isn't perfect, every day of his life now, he thanks Me for saving him from death and he tries his best to teach others about the love I have for everyone through my Son, Jesus Christ.

His soul was sick, dirty and broken and I restored it when He came and confessed His sins to me. I transformed Anthony's life. Will you be next?

Your Loving Father,
God

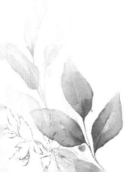

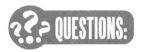 **QUESTIONS:**

1. How are you going to allow God to transform your life like He did to me?
2. How are you going to build a relationship with God?
3. How are you going to restore your relationship with God?

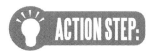 **ACTION STEP:**

1. If you're already baptized, go to google and type "Examination of Conscience" Click on the first link and reflect on the ten commandments. Go to your local church, confess your sins to a priest and head to weekly Eucharistic Mass and weekly Eucharistic Adoration. Email me if you are stuck or need help coachanthonysimon@gmail.com

27

Help! I'm Addicted & Ashamed

aving sex until marriage isn't just about saying no to temptation or sin, it's about saying yes to loving God and your future spouse. I know what you're thinking: "What about my need for sex? I'm addicted. How will I get that need met without sleeping with my boyfriend or girlfriend?" Okay, let me tell you how to get your sexual needs met while waiting until marriage. Are you ready?

THE BEAUTIFUL LIE: SEX IS A NEED

Sex is not a need. Your "sex needs" aren't on the to-do bucket list because sex is not a need. You don't need sex. You need comfort, intimacy, and connection—that's it. If you accept what your real needs are, your other "needs" (such as physical desires) will calm down and seem less demanding.

> You don't need sex. You need comfort, intimacy, and connection— that's it.

Take care of the basics first. If you get your soul and spirit needs met, your "physical needs" will diminish. The reason you can be so sex-obsessed and aroused all the time is because you aren't catering to your real needs. When you don't get these basic needs met in a healthy way, you get home and do something stupid like look at porn or hook up with your ex "one last time." You have starved yourself to the point where you will be satisfied with whatever is around. This is why when you're hungry, agitated, bored, anxious, lonely, or tired (H.A.B.A.L.T.), you want to engage in impurity.

So, the next time you're thinking about doing something sexual, ask yourself, "What do I need? Am I feeling truly connected to people in my life? How's my heart doing? Am I just stressed out about something? Am I lonely? Have I been vulnerable with people lately? Have I had a good workout? Am I tired? Am I bored?" When you're satisfied on the inside with good things, undesirable things won't look so enticing.

> **Intimacy is allowing someone to see you as you, love you for you, and value you for your uniqueness.**

There are many other ways to experience intimacy than just sex. Intimacy has been broken down like this by many: in-to-me-you-see. Intimacy is allowing someone to see you as you, love you for you, and value you for your uniqueness. You can only love to the extent that you're willing to be hurt. The deeper you let someone in, the bigger the risk is and the bigger the reward will be.

What do you turn to when it's late and you're tired, wanting comfort and a release of stress? Sex. Porn? Masturbation? Phone call with an ex? A shallow hookup? Why? It provides the necessary pleasure and comfort that your body is seeking, including feelings of security and peace. It's not meeting your truest needs of the soul (rest, safety, comfort), but it's an adequate, short-sighted solution (except for the side effects of shame, guilt, disconnection, and addiction).

If you're struggling with your sex drive, do a physical checkup: Are you eating well? Are you drinking enough water? Getting sunlight? Sleeping enough (eight hours of good quality sleep)? Are you getting enough healthy touch?

FEELING ASHAMED?

Don't let your past dictate your future. Jesus is always there whenever you are ready to earn back your trophy. He can restore anything with His mercy and grace. As crazy as it sounds, I've heard of people's virginities literally being restored. Again, it's not about being a virgin or not, but it's about being pure in heart, mind, and body. Virginity is just a fruit of purity. You could have the greatest past, but Jesus says, "I died for you on the cross to claim that past as My own so that you can have a future with Me. All I need you to do is acknowledge your mistakes, tell them to Me, and genuinely say you're sorry. There are always consequences to actions, but if you're truly sorry, I can alleviate the pain you feel. I am your comforter and I can restore everything for you. I just need you to believe. There is no circumstance I can't change, no amount of brokenness I can't heal, and no list of people you've slept with forged in your brain that I can't permanently erase from your memory. All you need to do is leave all your baggage at the foot of the cross. Give it to Me. Just try your best not to do it again. You've really got to show Me you're serious about changing, and I will erase every mistake as white as snow."

WHAT ABOUT SAFE SEX? (THE STATISTICS ABOUT SEX)

I made sure to put this extra section at the end of the book because it should be your least motivation to wait for sex until marriage, since it's a negative motivation out of fear that only focuses on the problems.

While condom use may reduce the risk of some sexually transmitted diseases, it doesn't offer much protection from HPV, because the virus is spread by skin-to-skin contact throughout the entire genital area, including one's thighs and lower abdomen.[1] The Centers for Disease Control reported that the majority of sexually active women have bene infected with one or more types of genital HPV.[2]

Doesn't sound so safe anymore, now,does it?

Still not convinced?

By having sexual contact with one person, you could be exposing yourself to the STDs of hundreds of people.[3] If you have sex with a person, you're basically having sex with everyone he or she had sex with, not to mention the others their partners have had sex with. It doesn't help that research also supports that 80 percent of people who have an STD are unaware of their own infections.[4]

I have talked to someone who was later married and thought they got away from the consequences of getting diseases because they practiced "safe sex" in the past. Several years later, however, the person was diagnosed with the HIV virus and showed symptoms of AIDS. Oral sex can transmit virtually every STD,[5] and hand-to-genital contact can transmit some as well.[6] So even virgins can get STDs,[7] including HPV, which can lead to oral cancer.[8]

If a woman gets chlamydia and isn't treated in time, she may become infertile. Seventy-five percent of women (and 50 percent of men) don't show symptoms after they contract it.[9] This is why it's called the "the silent sterilizer." Is it really worth getting into a relationship if you risk losing your ability to have kids?

Most STDs can be carried into marriage undetected. For example, 90 percent of people with genital herpes do not know that they are infected.[10] In the case of HPV, it will often clear up on its own. But when a husband is infected with it, his wife is five times as likely to get cervical cancer.[11] Several STDs are incurable, and many can be passed on from a mother to her baby, causing complications for the newborn such as brain damage, blindness, deafness, pneumonia, liver disease, and even death. If you want to know more about the statistics, check out Jason Evert's book *Pure Love*. It's only fifty pages and it's such an inspiration and quick read.

Ironic the world calls it "safe sex" because it's everything but safe. We need to protect the WHOLE person—not just their body, but the heart, soul, and spirit. Safe sex is very selfish in that it gives the permission to use others and lust over them instead of love over them. They live for the pleasures of sex without any lifelong commitment.

Your body, like your heart, isn't made for multiple sexual partners. It's made for enduring love.

Society is only pretending to solve your problems by using words that trigger your trust and safety responses. Realize this is a business at the end of the day, run by thirsty, money-sucking vampires that'll latch on to your life for their own selfish motives.

I don't believe in luck because luck is for leprechauns and you're not green.

Everyone likes to think that they are the exception. I find myself doing it all the time. But how can you control something that's uncontrollable? You can sit and justify all day long, but why even take the risk? Don't say, "I'm blessed" or "I got luck on my side." Let me tell you something about luck. I don't believe in luck because luck is for leprechauns and you're not green. Also, why test God? God isn't limited to just probabilities. He can do anything he wants at any time. Even if something is a 0.0000001 percent chance of happening, He can make it into a 100 percent chance of happening so that you can potentially learn from your mistakes.

I mean, at the end of the day, when I read information like this and see all the problems, I start to understand why God really doesn't want us having any form of sex before marriage and that there are consequences for disregarding His teachings. It's such a holy way of showing God's love. No wonder the enemy tries to manipulate it the hardest. He wants to rob you of authentic love. Don't fall for his beautiful lies and traps now that you know better.

You weren't designed to give pieces of yourself. You were designed to give all of yourself.

You weren't designed to give pieces of yourself. You were designed to give all of yourself. You weren't designed to give 50 percent of your commitment; you were designed to give 100 percent of your commitment, which is why when a child is born, they say, "Mama. Dada. Hello. You two are in charge of me. I need 100 percent commitment from the both of you, otherwise I will have problems."

Listen to what God has to say about sex. This is the final chapter of His own love letter to you, which summarizes why He too instructs us to wait until marriage to have sex and practice purity of mind and heart.

GOD'S FINAL LOVE LETTER

My Precious Child,

You have reached the final chapter of my own love letter to you. I'm so proud of you.

So, now you know that My son wants to restore your purity according to how I envisioned it to be. Through My love and mercy and following My commandments you can do so, but there is a problem: Every human being is born with weakened wills, disordered appetites, and darkened intellects. This inclination to sin is called concupiscence. It is what constantly pushes you to cross the boundary between passively feeling temptation and actively choosing it.

Because of original sin, you do not rule over your body and passions, so you must learn how to conquer your passions with discipline and self-control. Many people give up because they are addicted to the pleasure and don't know how to change. Instead of seeing love as the motivation behind no sex until marriage, you see Me as a tyrant and a holdout.

FEELING ADDICTED?

Now do you see why I said put to death sexual immortality, impurity, lust, evil desires, and greed, which is idolatry? (Colossians 3:5). You can easily become addicted, for as a dog returns to its vomit, so fools repeat their sins (Proverbs 26:11).

You know that it is My will that you should be sanctified; that you should avoid sexual immorality and that you should learn to control your own body in a way that is holy and honorable (1 Thessalonians

4:3-4). You know I have not called you to be impure but to live a holy life (1 Thessalonians 4:7) by keeping the marriage bed pure for your one and only spouse (Hebrews 13:4). I have asked you to not awaken love until marriage (Song of Songs 2:7) but some of you choose not to listen to Me you have become addicted and slaves to your own passions and desires. Some of you didn't know better or let pressure get to you so you conformed to the patterns of this world. (Romans 12:2) Lastly, some of you have been victims of sexual abuse. In this case, allow Me to use it for your good and perfectly heal you.

When you sin sexually, it's the only sin in which you sin against your own body; this is why I asked you to flee from sexual immorality. Your body is a temple of the Holy Spirit who is in you, who you received from Me. Your body isn't yours, it's Mine. Therefore, honor Me with your body (1 Corinthians 6:18-20).

I know you do not understand what you do for what you want to do you do not do, but what you hate you do. Understand that it is the sinful nature from Adam and Eve that you have grown living in you causing you to do what you don't want to do. Your flesh and spirit are waging war, causing you to not do the good you want to do, but to continue to do evil. You say you are a slave to sin but I say something else (Romans 7). I say I have conquered and defeated sin by My death and resurrection. Overcome sin too by receiving the sacrament confession. When you're baptized, your old self will be crucified with Me so that your body rules by sin might be done away with; you shall no longer be a slave to sin. You have been set free from your sins and your sins should no longer be your master, because you will be under My grace and sin shall have no dominion over you (Romans 6). So, come boldly to My throne of grace in the sacrament of confession, so that you may obtain mercy and find My grace to help you in times of need and temptation (Hebrews 4:16).

CAN I REALLY DO THIS? NOBODY ELSE IS

I do not command that which cannot be done.

Do not be conformed to the patterns of this world (Romans 12:2). If the world hates you, keep in mind that it hated Me first. If you belonged to the world, it would love you as its own. As it is, you do not belong to the world, but I have chosen you out of the world. That is why the world hates you (John 15:18-19). When your flesh and your heart fail, know I am the strength of your heart (Psalm 73:26). You then, My child, be strong in the grace that is in Christ Jesus (2 Timothy 2:1).

- You say: I can't figure it out. I say: I will direct your steps (Proverbs 3:5-6)
- You say: I'm too tired. I say: I will give you rest (Matthew 11:28-30)
- You say: It's impossible. I say: All things are possible (Luke 18:27)
- You say: Nobody loves me. I say: I love you. (John 3:16)
- You say: I can't forgive myself. I say: I forgive you. (Romans 8:1)
- You say: It's not worth it. I say: It will be worth it. (Romans 8:28)
- You say: I'm not smart enough. I say: I will give you wisdom. (1 Corinthians 12:9)
- You say: I'm not able. I say: You are able. (2 Corinthians 9:8)
- You say: I can't go on. I say: My grace is sufficient. (2 Corinthians 12:9)
- You say: I can't do it. I say: You can do all things through me. (Philippians 4:13)
- You say: I can't manage. I say: I will supply all your needs. (Philippians 4:19)
- You say: I'm afraid. I say: I have not given you fear. (2 Timothy 1:7)
- You say: I feel all alone. I say: I will never leave you. (Hebrews 13:5)

Look, My child. All I'm trying to get you to understand is that your physician who has the title "doctor" isn't your doctor. I am your doctor. I am your counselor. I am your coach. I am your provider. I am your cheerleader. I am your loving Father. Let Me restore you. Let Me teach you. I know you're hurting and trying everything under the sun to cure your loneliness you've had your whole life, but how much suffering are you going to endure until you learn that I am the solution to all of your problems? It breaks My heart to see you in pain, but I have to allow it because it's the only way to not only turn your head but also turn your heart and show you that I am God. I am who I say I am. I am your source of happiness. It's okay to be lonely sometimes, but come to Me first. Don't go out to others to heal your loneliness. Just say to Me, "God, I am sick and tired of being sick and tired," and I will take you as My child, for I am the provider of all graces and mercies, the one who will turn your shameful scars to sacred scars to heal others. You need only to trust who I say I am. I am God. Do you trust Me?

I love you. Please don't stop with just this book. Continue to develop a relationship with Me and seek Me with all your heart. I am waiting for you. How much longer will you keep Me waiting? How many more times will I continue chasing you? How much longer my child? How much longer?

Your Loving Father,
The Almighty God

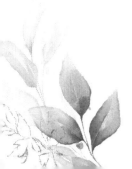

236

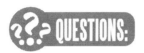

QUESTIONS:

1. What have you learned throughout this book? What did you like? (Bonus points if you leave a review telling me on Amazon!)
2. How can you develop a greater relationship with God?
3. Do you have any questions for me? I'm an open book, as you can tell, and I genuinely want to hear your story.

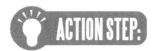

ACTION STEP:

1. Review your journal notes on my book. Then, take a picture with my book, leave a review on my Amazon page with your favorite notes. Share your story and lessons learned with others so they can be inspired too. Feel free to even leave a video review on my amazon page. Message me at coachanthonysimon@gmail.com when you finished.

CONCLUSION

I love you.

No seriously. I love you from the depths of my heart.

Don't believe me? Let my actions speak louder than my words. Publishing this book was a huge risk. I most certainly will lose friends, be laughed at, mocked, and persecuted for releasing this book. The sacrifices I've made for this book were unreal. This book wasn't supposed to be published, but in the end, God gave me the green light. Even though I may look like a fool in the world's eyes for releasing this book, I want you to know one thing . . . I love you.

I'm going to meet God face to face one day and He will ask me, "Son, did you share my love with others? Did you make the love I've shown you known?" I can't imagine meeting God face to face and telling him I was too scared to release this book because of the opinions of others. You're worth more than my fears, insecurities, embarrassments, doubts, failures and persecutions. Your soul is far more precious to me than my reputation. I truly do love you and if you knew just how much I loved you, you would cry. I guarantee that.

Although I love you deeply, God loves you even more. I am only able to love you because He first loved me and my brokenness. When you see nothing in yourself, He sees something in you.

I STILL FEEL ASHAMED AND HOPELESS

If you're feeling ashamed or don't believe Jesus can ever restore your purity or forgive you because of your past, you're wrong. Jesus forgave St. Mary Magdalene who was known for sleeping around. She was genuinely sorry, got on her knees, and wiped Jesus's feet with her tears. If Jesus forgave her because of her sincerity to change her ways, why won't He forgive you? It's pride to think that He can't forgive you. Your past is not greater than His mercy. There are countless stories of Jesus's mercy and forgiveness. You need to only believe He is bigger than your past and trust in His love and mercy for you.

You may be saying, "Ok, Anthony I'm forgiven. What about my stickiness you were talking about in chapter 10? What about the brain chemistry in Chapter 9? What about my ability to love my future spouse? Am I less because of my past?"

I'll answer by this simple question. Do you not believe in the power of God? Is science greater than God the almighty? Why limit Jesus and His power to statistics? He is the almighty who can do all things. He helped me write this book and that was a miracle in itself. God transformed my life. I never knew I'd ever be a writer or a speaker. They were my two greatest weaknesses. I didn't start reading a book until I was 19 years old. I had public speaking anxiety and a stuttering problem. But let me tell you something about my God. He's not a religion, He's a lifestyle. My God breathes. He lives. He speaks. Most importantly my God forgives. He turns our mistakes and greatest weakness to our greatest strengths. He's your God too if you make Him. If you don't believe me, listen to Jesus's very own words to St. Margaret of Cortona who had the same questions as you.

Jesus Christ: My daughter, one day I will place you among the Seraphs, among the virgins whose hearts are flaming with love for God.

St. Margaret of Cortona: How can that be, Lord, after I have soiled myself with so many sins?

Jesus Christ: My daughter, your many penances have purified your soul from all the effects of sin to such a degree that your contrition and your sufferings will reintegrate you *into the purity of a virgin.*

Listen.

Jesus's greatest saints that have ever lived were His greatest sinners. You can be one of the holiest people to ever walk in this planet if you just trust in the mercy of God. You have the ability to love deeper than me and other virgins in this world when you experience the mercy and love of God. That's not to say it's going to be a great challenge to overcome, but it is to say that *when* you do experience God's mercy and overcome your past through God's grace, you will understand love much deeper than I ever will. Therefore, you will have the greatest relationship ever.

I believe in you. Anything is possible if you set your mind to it and believe with all your heart that God has got your back and will restore you fully. If her purity and virginity was restored physically, yours can be too. St. Margaret of Cortona's story is one of many. I have heard countless stories of people's purities and even virginities being restored fully. Not only experience attests to this, but science does too. When you practice purity, your brain chemistry readjusts. This goes to show God's mercy. It's never too late. Today is *YOUR* day. Are you ready to begin this new journey?

Man. This has been quite the journey with you and I hope you feel inspired to wait until marriage now to have sex. If I am a twenty-two-year-old virgin who survived college without sex because of God's grace, you should be able to wait until marriage too. Lots of people like me exist. Believe me. We're just all scattered so we can be the light to our cities' darkness.

RESOURCES:

I want to provide you with the community, prayers and resources to stand firm in your vision. If you're ever feeling alone, just find other communities that help build your vision up and support you. Heck, you have me but there are a whole bunch of us. Check out Jason Evert and the Chastity Project. I don't want to overload you but start there.

Ask for the intercession of these particular saints to pray for you who are well known for chastity and purity.

1. St. Joseph
2. St. Mary Magdalene
3. St. Maria Goretti
4. St. Margaret of Cortona
5. The Blessed Virgin Mary

When you fail . . . don't beat yourself up. Head to the sacrament of confession and confess your sins to a priest. You're not going to be perfect but just never stop striving for perfection.

Again, I love you dearly. I want to hear back from you not only when you find your future spouse and thank me for waiting, but also right now. If you enjoyed our journey together, please head to Amazon to leave a review for my book. It'll help other readers know what to expect, so I can reach the widest audience possible. Let's stay connected. I want to hear your story. Reach out to me by email at coachanthonysimon@ gmail.com and don't forget to leave a review for me on Amazon.

I want to close off with a prayer that changed my life.

LITANY OF TRUST

From the belief that I have to earn Your love

Deliver me, Jesus.

From the fear that I am unlovable

Deliver me, Jesus.

From the false security that I have what it takes

Deliver me, Jesus.

From the fear that trusting You will leave me more destitute

Deliver me, Jesus.

From all suspicion of Your words and promises

Deliver me, Jesus.

From the rebellion against childlike dependency on You

Deliver me, Jesus.

From refusals and reluctances in accepting Your will

Deliver me, Jesus.

From anxiety about the future

Deliver me, Jesus.

From resentment or excessive preoccupation with the past

Deliver me, Jesus.

From restless self-seeking in the present moment

Deliver me, Jesus.

From disbelief in Your love and presence

Deliver me, Jesus.

From the fear of being asked to give more than I have

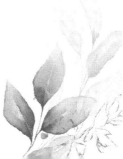

Deliver me, Jesus.

From the belief that my life has no meaning or worth

Deliver me, Jesus.

From the fear of what love demands

Deliver me, Jesus.

From discouragement

Deliver me, Jesus.

That You are continually holding me, sustaining me, loving me

Jesus, I trust in You.

That Your love goes deeper than my sins and failings and transforms me

Jesus, I trust in You.

That not knowing what tomorrow brings is an invitation to lean on You

Jesus, I trust in You.

That You are with me in my suffering

Jesus, I trust in You.

That my suffering, united to Your own, will bear fruit in this life and the next

Jesus, I trust in You.

That You will not leave me orphan, that You are present in Your Church

Jesus, I trust in You.

That Your plan is better than anything else

Jesus, I trust in You.

That You always hear me and in Your goodness always respond to me

Jesus, I trust in You.

That You give me the grace to accept forgiveness and to forgive others

Jesus, I trust in You.

That You give me all the strength I need for what is asked

Jesus, I trust in You.

That my life is a gift

Jesus, I trust in You.

That You will teach me to trust You

Jesus, I trust in You.

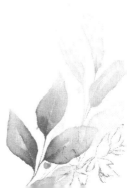

ABOUT THE AUTHOR

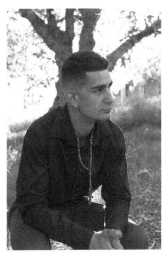

Anthony Simon is a professional motivational speaker, #1 bestselling author, life coach, and CEO of Coach Anthony Simon who graduated from the University of California, Davis, with degrees in Bio-Psychology (B.S.) and Communications (B.A.). Speaking and empowering over ten thousand people, Anthony travels around the U.S., coaching youth and young adults in mind, body, and spirit through social emotional learning. Anthony is known for informing and inspiring his audience to live in sustaining happiness and unconditional love. At twenty-one, as a student-athlete and double major, Anthony published the #1 best-selling book, Life's Greatest Gift: P.A.I.N., that ranked in the top 1 percent out of 9 million books on Amazon.

Motivational, inspirational and always approachable, Anthony is deeply passionate for the personal development of students, youth and young adults through social emotional learning. Anthony's tell-it-like-it-is attitude is a refreshing approach that allows him to authentically connect with his audience in a heartfelt, informative and inspirational way. He wants the next generation to live up to his slogan, "Love Your Life." Anthony Simon currently lives in Sacramento, California.

For more information about Anthony visit:
www.coachanthonysimon.com

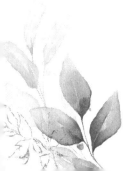

NOTES

Chapter 9

1. Mcllhaney, Joe s., and Freda Mckissic Bush. Hooked: New Science on How Casual Sex Is Affecting Our Children. Chicago: Northfield Pub., 2008. Print. 45.
2. Ibid., 16
3. Ibid., 33
4. Carmichael, et al., "Plasma oxytocin increases in the human sexual response," *The Journal of Clinical Endocrinology and Metabolism* 64:1 (January 1987): 27-31; Murphy, et al., "Changes in Oxytocin and vasopressin secretion during sexual activity in men," *The Journal of Clinical Endocrinology and Metabolism* 65:4 (October 1987): 738-741.
5. Kosfeld, et al., "Oxytocin increases trust in humans," *Nature* 435 (2005): 673-676; Heinrichs, et al., "Selective Amnesic effects of oxytocin on human memory," *Physiology & Behavior 83 (2004):* 31-38; Bartz, et al., "the neuroscience of affiliation: Foreign links between basic and clinical research on neuropeptides and social behavior." *Hormones and Behavior* 50 (2006): 518-528; B. Ditzen, "Effects of Social Support and Oxytocin on Psychological and Physiological Stress Responses during Marital conflict," International Congress

of Neuroendocrinology, Pittsburgh, PA: June 19-22, 2006; Crenshaw, M.D., *The Alchemy of Love and Lust* (New York: Pocket Books, 1996)

6. Bartels and Zeki, "The neural correlates of maternal and romantic love," *NeuroImage* 21 (2004): 1155-1166

7. Cf. Pfaff, et al., "Neural Oxytocinergic Systems as Genomic Targets for Hormones and as Modulators of Hormone-Dependent Behaviors," *Results and Problems in Cell Differentiation* 26 (1999): 91-105, as quoted by Eric J. Keroack, M.D., and John R. Diggs, Jr., M.D., "Bonding Imperative," A Special Report from the Abstinence Medical Council (Abstinence Clearinghouse, April 30, 2001): K. Joyner and R. Udry, "You Don't Bring Me Anything but Down: Adolescent Romance and Depression," *Journal of Health and social Behavior* 41:4 (December 2000): 361-391: Hallfors, et al., "Which Comes first in Adolescence—Sex and Drugs or Depression?" *American Journal of Preventive Medicine* 29:3 (2005): 163-170.

8. Mcllhaney, Joe s., and Freda Mckissic Bush. Hooked: New Science on How Casual Sex Is Affecting Our Children. Chicago: Northfield Pub., 2008. Print. 38

9. Ibid., 32

Chapter 10

1. Mcllhaney, Joe s., and Freda Mckissic Bush. Hooked: New Science on How Casual Sex Is Affecting Our Children. Chicago: Northfield Pub., 2008. Print. 43

2. "New Marriage and Divorce Statistics Released." The Barna Group, 31 Mar. 2008. Web. <https://www.barna.org/family-kids-articles/42-new-marriage-and-divorce-statistics-released, March, 2008>.

Chapter 11

1. Cf. William R. Mattox, Jr., "Aha! Call it the revenge of the church ladies," USA TODAY, February 11,1999, 15-A.
2. Cf. William R. Mattox Jr., "The Hottest Valentines: the Startling Secret of What Makes You a High-Voltage Lover," The Washington Post, February 13, 1994

Chapter 22

1. Doige,Norman. "BrianScansofPornAddicts."TheGuardian,26Sept, 2013. Web. <Http://www.theguardian.com/commentisfree/2013/ sep/26/brain-scans-porn-addicts-sexual-tastes>

Chapter 27

1. Cf. National Institutes of Health, "Scientific Evidence on Condom Effectiveness for Sexually Transmitted Disease (STD) Prevention" (June 2000) 26, www.niaid.nih.gov/dmid/ stds/codomreport.pdf; House of Representatives, "Breast and Cervical Cancer Prevention and Treatment Act of 1999," November 22,1999.
2. Division of STD Prevention, "Prevention of Genital HPV Infection and Sequelae: Report of an External Consultants' Meeting," 7.
3. Cf. Bearman, et al., "Chains of Affection: The Structure of Adolescent Romantic Sexual Networks," *American Journal of Sociology* 110:1 (2004): 44-91
4. Joe McIlhaney, M.D., *Safe Sex* (Grand Rapids, MI: Baker Book House, 1991), 23.
5. Cf. Medical "Institute for Sexual Health, *Sex, Condoms, and STDs*: What we now Know (Austin, TX: Medical Institute for Sexual Health, 2002); B. Dillion, "Primary HIV Infections Associated with Oral Transmission," CDC's 7th Conference

on Retroviruses and Opportunistic Infection, Abstract 473, San Francisco, February 2000; Centers for Disease Control, "Transmission of Primary and Secondary Syphilis by Oral Sex—Chicago, Illinois 1998-2002," *Morbidity and Mortality Weekly Report* 51:41 (October 22,2004): 966-968.

6. Cf. C, Sonnex, et al., "Detection of Human Papillomavirus DNA on the Fingers of Patients with Genital Warts," *Sexually Transmitted Infections* 75 (1999): 317-319; Winer, et al., "Genital Human Papillomavirus Infection: Incidence and Risk Factors in a Cohort of Female University Students," *American Journal of Epidemiology* 157:3 (2003): 218-226; Tabrizi, et al., "Prevalence of Gardnerella vaginalis and Atopobium vaginae in virginal women," *Journal of the National Clinical Microbiology & Infectious Diseases* 12:3 (March 1993): 221-223

7. Cf. Ley, et al., "Determinates of Genital Human Papillomavirus Infection in Young Women," *Journal of the National Cancer Institute* 83:14 (July 1991): 997-1003; Pao, et al., "Possible non-sexual transmission of genital human papillomavirus infections in young women," *European Journal of Clinical Microbiology & Infectious Diseases* 12:3 (March 1993): 221-223

8. Cf. Hammarstedt, et al., "Human papillomavirus as a risk factor for the increase in incidence of tonsillar cancer," *International Journal of Cancer* 119:11 (December 2006): 2620-2623.

9. Centers for Disease Control, "Tracking the Hidden Epidemics, Trends in STDs in the United States 2000," (April 6, 2001), 6.

10. Cf. P. Leone, "Type-specific Serologic Testing for Herpes Simplex Virus-2," *Current Infectious Disease Reports* 5:2 (April 2003): 159-165.

11. Cf. Bosch, et al., "Male Sexual Behavior and Human Papillomavirus DNA: Key Risk Factors for Cervical Cancer in Spain," *Journal of the National Cancer Institute* 88:15 (August 1996): 1060-1067

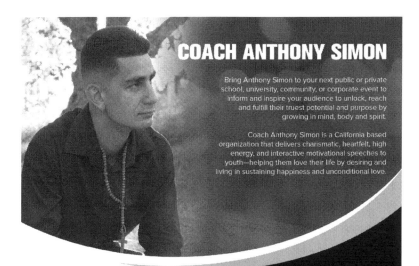
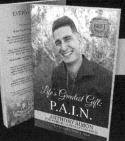

Made in the USA
San Bernardino, CA
08 July 2020